# HOW TO LOSE WEIGHT IN 30 DAYS

A PROVEN DAILY PLAN TO BURN FAT, TRANSFORM YOUR BODY, AND TAKE BACK CONTROL IN JUST 30 DAYS

INSPIRED LEGACY PRESS

EDGAR HERNÁNDEZ

INSPIRED
LEGACY PRESS

# COPYRIGHT



**Published by Inspired Legacy Press**

Sparks, Nevada, USA

**ISBN: 978-1-971513-20-1**

**Book Design and Layout:** Inspired Legacy Press

**Logo:** Inspired Enterprises LLC



**First Edition — 2025**

**Printed in the United States of America**

# EPIGRAPH

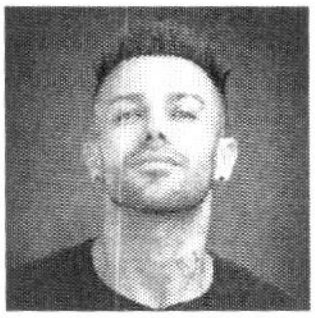

"The body does not change when you punish it.
It changes when you begin to respect it.
It responds exactly to the life you have been living.
Change your decisions... and your body will change with you."

— Edgar Hernández · Inspired Legacy Press

*Dedicated to those who have tried to start over again and again.*
*To those who grew tired of failing, but not of trying.*
*To those who know their body is not the enemy,*
*but a reflection of the choices they are now ready to change.*
*This book is for you.*

*— Edgar Hernández*

# ACKNOWLEDGMENTS

Thank you to every person who chose not to give up, even after failing.
To those who understood that true change does not begin in the body,
but in the decision to take responsibility for their life.
Thank you to the human body, for its infinite capacity to adapt, heal, and transform when it is given what it needs.
Thank you to discipline, time, and consistency, because they always tell the truth.
Thank you to knowledge, to science, and to real experience,
for proving that there are no lasting shortcuts—
only well-executed processes.
And thank you to you, holding this book in your hands.
If you are here, it is because you are ready to do things differently.
This is not the beginning of a diet—
it is the beginning of a new way of living in your body.

— Edgar Hernández

# CONTENTS

## IT'S NOT YOUR BODY.
## IT'S THE SYSTEM.

You didn't arrive at this book by accident.

You arrived because something inside you grew tired of half-hearted attempts—

of starting with enthusiasm and quitting with guilt,

of promising yourself "this time for real,"

only to end up in the same place months later.

And I want to tell you something from the very beginning, without detours:

Your body is not the problem.

It never was.

The body is honest. Precise. Relentlessly consistent.

It does nothing at random.

It does not betray you.

It does not conspire against you.

Your body responds exactly to the way you have lived, eaten, rested, thought,

and made decisions for years.

The problem is not a lack of willpower.

It is not your age.

It is not a "slow" metabolism.

It is not that you're "bad at dieting."

The real problem has always been the same:

you've tried to change results without changing the system.

For years, you were sold quick fixes, punishments disguised as discipline,

rules impossible to sustain, and plans that only work while you suffer through them.

You were told that to change your body, you had to fight it—

humiliate it, restrict it, exhaust it.

And every time you failed, the blame fell on you.

This book exists to break that cycle.

Here you will not find a miracle diet.

You will not find unrealistic promises or magic formulas.

You will not find punishment or extremes.

You will find something far more powerful:

A daily plan. Clear. Executable. Sustainable.

A system that works with your body, not against it.

A process that understands that real change does not happen in a day,

but it can begin today.

Over the next 30 days, I will not ask for perfection.

I will ask for presence.

I will not ask for heroic sacrifices.

I will ask for conscious decisions.

I will not ask you to become someone else.

I will help you become who you are already capable of being.

If you follow this plan, your body will change.

But more importantly,

your relationship with it will change.

You will learn to listen to real signals.

To build habits that do not depend on motivation.

To create results that do not require punishment to last.

This is not a book to start "over again."

It is a book to start right.

If you are willing to follow a simple, honest, and consistent process,

this will be the exact point where everything began to change.

Not because you tried harder—

but because, for the first time, you did it the right way.

Welcome.

The plan starts now.

# INTRODUCTION

This is not a book to read.
It is a book to do.

Before continuing, I need you to understand something with absolute clarity:

This book was not written to entertain you.

It was written to change what you do every day—

because that is the only thing that changes the body.

If you read it like any other book, nothing will happen.

If you consume it as just more information, nothing will happen.

If you are looking for temporary motivation, this is not your place.

But if you are willing to follow a plan—

even if it's simple,

even if it's uncomfortable at first,

even if it doesn't feel perfect—

then this book can become a real before and after in your life.

Most people don't fail because they don't know what to do.

They fail because they:

- try to change everything at once
- demand perfection from themselves
- depend on motivation
- quit when they don't see immediate results

This book was designed to eliminate those mistakes at the root.

Here you will not find unnecessary theory.

You will not find extreme rules.

You will not find a system that only works under ideal conditions.

You will find something far more valuable:

Structure.

A daily plan that tells you:

- what to do
- what to focus on
- what to avoid
- and how to move forward without burning out

Over the next 30 days, you won't have to guess anything.

You won't have to improvise.

You won't have to rely on infinite willpower.

You will only have to follow the day you're on.

This book was created for real men and women.

With jobs.

With stress.

With fatigue.

With history.

With failed attempts.

**You don't need to be motivated to start.**
**You need to be committed to continuing.**
**And here is the most important part:**
**Don't chase fast results.**
**Chase real results.**
**Because when you do the right things consistently, the body responds.**
**It always does.**
**If you follow this plan:**

- your energy will change
- your relationship with food will change
- your body will begin to transform
- and your mind will stop sabotaging you

**Not because you did something extreme, but because you did the right things for long enough.**
**This is not the beginning of a diet.**
**It is the beginning of a system.**
**Read each day with intention.**
**Execute with honesty.**
**Move forward without rush—but without pause.**
**Change does not begin tomorrow.**
**It does not begin on Monday.**
**It does not begin when you "have time."**
**It begins now.**
**Turn the page.**
**Day 1 is waiting for you.**

# PART I

# PREPARATION

Before changing the body, the mind must be prepared.

Before we talk about plans, days, actions, or results, there is something that must be absolutely clear:

There is no physical transformation without mental preparation.

Not because the body is complicated, but because the mind is often the first obstacle.

Misunderstood beliefs, past experiences, accumulated frustration, and unrealistic expectations cause many people to quit before they even begin.

This first part of the book exists to clear the path.

You will not find daily instructions here yet.

This is not the time to measure, adjust, or demand results from yourself.

This is the time to understand.

To understand:

- why your body works the way it does
- why what you tried before didn't last
- and which rules actually produce real change

Most people enter a weight-loss process in a hurry.

They want immediate results, quick signals, constant confirmation.

That urgency is often the beginning of abandonment.

This section will help you slow down your mind—not your commitment.

To stop fighting your body.

To stop blaming yourself for past failures.

To understand that you didn't lack discipline—you lacked structure.

When you understand the process, anxiety decreases.

When anxiety decreases, consistency increases.

And when consistency appears, results stop being a mystery.

Part 1 is intentionally brief.

It is not a theoretical course.

It is a calibration.

Read it calmly.

Don't underline to memorize.

Underline to understand.

When you finish this section, you will not feel motivated.

You will feel aligned.

And that is far more powerful.

Starting in the next chapter, we will begin dismantling myths, clarifying truths, and establishing the rules that will make the next 30 days work the way they should.

**Do not move forward in a rush.**
**Move forward with intention.**
**The body will change later.**
**First, let's prepare the mind.**

# 1

# THE TRUTH ABOUT WEIGHT LOSS

Most people believe that losing weight is a matter of willpower.

That those who succeed are more disciplined, stronger, or simply "better" than those who don't.

That idea is false.

And it is one of the main reasons so many people fail again and again.

Losing weight is not an act of force.

It is a consequence.

A direct consequence of how you eat, how you move, how you rest, how you manage stress,

and—above all—the decisions you repeat every day.

The body does not respond to promises.

It does not respond to emotions.

It does not respond to guilt or intention.

It responds to patterns.

If you have lived a certain way for years, your body simply adapted to that.

It did not punish you.

It did not betray you.

It did exactly what it needed to do to survive under those conditions.

That is why, when someone tries to change their body without changing their lifestyle system,

the result is usually the same: intense effort, temporary results, and an inevitable return to the starting point.

Not because the body "rebounds,"

but because it returns to the environment it knows.

The most common mistake

The mistake is not wanting to lose weight.

The mistake is trying to do it through punishment.

Extreme diets.

Impossible restrictions.

Routines that don't fit real life.

Plans that only work while you suffer through them.

That approach creates two serious problems:

1 It is not sustainable

2 It breaks your relationship with your body

When something feels like punishment, it is eventually abandoned.

And when it is abandoned, guilt appears.

And when guilt appears, the body is treated as the enemy once again.

This book exists to break that cycle.

The truth almost no one talks about

The body does not need to be dominated.

It needs to be understood.

You don't need to eat less until you disappear.

You need to eat better—with structure.

You don't need to train until exhaustion.

You need to move consistently.

You don't need endless motivation.

You need habits that work even when you don't feel like it.

When you do the right things consistently, the body responds.

It always responds.

Not in one day.

Not in one week.

But it responds.

And when it does, it does so in a logical, progressive, and measurable way.

Real results vs. fast results

Fast results are often impressive... and fragile.

Real results are quieter—but they last.

This book was not designed to help you lose weight as fast as possible.

It was designed to help you never gain it back.

That changes everything.

Here, you will not fight your body.

You will align with it.

You will learn to:

- create an environment that makes good decisions easier
- reduce friction in your daily life
- eliminate extremes
- and build cumulative progress

You don't need to change everything today.

You need to start changing something... and sustain it.

What you need to remember from this point forward

Burn this into your mind before moving on:

- Your body is not broken
- You are not lacking discipline
- You didn't fail because you couldn't

- You failed because you didn't have a system

**That ends here.**

**In the next chapters, we will dismantle the most common myths, establish clear rules,**

**and prepare the ground for the 30-day plan that comes next.**

**Do not move forward looking for miracles.**

**Move forward looking for coherence.**

**When there is coherence between what you do and what your body needs,**

**the body has no choice but to change.**

**And now that you know the truth,**

**it's time to move forward.**

# 2

# WHY MOST PEOPLE FAIL (AND YOU WON'T)

Most people don't fail because they don't want to change.

They fail because they try to change the wrong way.

If you've ever started with enthusiasm, done "everything right" for a few days or weeks,

and then quit, it wasn't a lack of character.

It was a lack of structure.

You are not the problem.

The approach is.

The failure cycle

Almost everyone follows the same pattern:

1 They get tired of how they look or feel

2 They promise themselves "this time for real"

3 They start all-in

4 They demand perfection

5 They burn out

6 They quit

7 They blame themselves

8 They repeat the cycle months later

This cycle doesn't happen because of weakness.

It happens because it's built on invisible mistakes.

Mistake #1: Trying to change everything at once

Changing your food, exercise, schedule, sleep, routine, mindset, and entire life all at once

is a guaranteed recipe for burnout.

The body and mind don't change through explosions of effort.

They change through manageable consistency.

When you try to do everything perfectly from day one,

any mistake feels like total failure.

And when everything feels like failure, quitting feels logical.

This book eliminates that mistake from the very beginning.

Mistake #2: Depending on motivation

Motivation is unstable.

It rises when you feel inspired and disappears when you're tired, stressed, or busy.

If your progress depends on motivation,

your progress will be inconsistent.

People who achieve real change aren't the most motivated.

They're the ones with a system that works even on bad days.

Here, you won't depend on motivation.

You'll depend on structure.

Mistake #3: Confusing sacrifice with progress

For years, we were taught that if it doesn't hurt, it doesn't work.

That extreme exhaustion is a sign of progress.

That suffering is part of the process.

That's not only false—it's dangerous.

Real progress feels sustainable, not destructive.

Challenging, but doable.

Demanding, but compatible with real life.

When something feels like punishment,

the body and mind look for an escape.

And they always find one.

Mistake #4: Chasing fast results

The urgency to see immediate change pushes many people

to make decisions they can't sustain.

They eat too little.

They train too much.

They sleep poorly.

They ignore their body's signals.

The result may be rapid weight loss...

almost always followed by an equal or greater rebound.

Not because the body is traitorous,

but because it protects its balance.

This book wasn't designed to impress in a week.

It was designed to work over time.

Mistake #5: Believing the past defines the future

Many people carry a dangerous internal story:

"I always quit."

"It's harder for me."

"I've already tried everything."

Those statements don't describe who you are.

They describe what you did without structure.

The past doesn't prove inability.

It proves you hadn't yet found the right method for you.

Why you won't fail

You won't fail for one simple reason:

This book doesn't ask for perfection.

It asks for consistency.

It doesn't ask you to change your life.

It asks you to follow a clear daily plan.

It doesn't ask you to be strong.

It gives you structure to move forward even when you're tired.

There are no punishments here.

No extremes.

No impossible rules.

Only small decisions, repeated with intention.

And that changes everything.

From this point on, stop measuring progress by emotions.

Measure it by executed actions.

One day completed.

Another day completed.

Another one.

That is real progress.

And now that you understand why most people fail, you're ready to learn the rules that actually work.

# 3

# THE RULES OF THE GAME: WHAT ACTUALLY WORKS

If you've made it this far, you already understand something fundamental:

your body doesn't need punishment—it needs coherence.

Now it's time to establish the rules of the game.

Not extreme rules.

Not perfect rules.

Real rules, designed to work in everyday life.

These rules are not meant to control you.

They are meant to free you from confusion.

Rule #1: Consistency matters more than intensity

Doing a little every day beats doing a lot only when you have energy.

The body changes when it receives consistent signals,

not when it receives sporadic bursts of effort.

One good decision repeated one hundred times

is worth more than one perfect decision made once.

You won't win here through intensity.

You'll win through continuity.

Rule #2: Progress is built, not improvised

Improvisation is the enemy of change.

When you don't know what to do, you choose what's easiest.

When you choose what's easiest every day, the body responds to that.

That's why this book gives you a daily plan.

Not to control you, but to eliminate mental friction.

Fewer unnecessary decisions.

More execution.

Rule #3: The body responds to habits, not emotions

You may feel motivated today and exhausted tomorrow.

The body doesn't care.

The body responds to:

- what you eat consistently
- how you move regularly
- how you rest
- how you manage stress

Emotions change.

Habits stay.

This process does not depend on feeling good.

It depends on doing the right thing even when it's uncomfortable.

Rule #4: What's sustainable always wins

If you can't maintain it, it doesn't count.

Any strategy you can't sustain for months

is destined to fail—even if it works at first.

That's why here:

- there are no extremes
- there are no absurd prohibitions
- there are no unnecessary sacrifices

The goal is not to lose weight fast.

The goal is not to gain it back.

**Rule #5: The body needs time, not pressure**

The body doesn't negotiate with urgency.

It negotiates with consistency.

Pressure creates resistance.

Support creates change.

When you give the body what it needs for long enough,

it responds.

It always responds.

**Rule #6: Environment matters more than willpower**

Relying on willpower alone is a weak strategy.

Your environment determines:

- what you eat
- how much you move
- how you rest
- how easy or difficult it is to follow through

This book will help you create an environment

that works in your favor—not against you.

**Rule #7: Not all change is immediately visible**

At first, some changes are felt before they're seen:

- more energy
- better sleep
- less anxiety
- greater mental clarity

That is progress too.

The mistake is quitting because "it doesn't show yet."

The win is continuing because something is already being built.

**Rule #8: The system is stronger than any excuse**

When you have a clear system, excuses lose their power.

You don't need motivation.

You need to follow the day you're on.

**A well-designed system overcomes fatigue, stress, and difficult days.**

**And that is exactly what comes next.**

**Before moving forward**

**Remember this:**

- You are not starting a diet
- You are entering a process
- You are not fighting your body
- You are learning to work with it

**The preparation is complete.**

**The rules are clear.**

**The mind is aligned.**

**Now—yes.**

**On the next page, the 30-Day Plan begins.**

**This is where everything turns into action.**

**Breathe.**

**Commit.**

**And take the first step.**

## PART II

# THE 30-DAY PLAN

This is where the work gets done.

Up to this point, you've understood something fundamental:

change doesn't happen by trying harder—it happens by doing things better.

Now we leave theory behind.

You're not here to reflect.

You're here to act.

Part 2 of this book is the core of the entire process.

It's not a reading experience.

It's a daily execution plan.

Over the next 30 days, you won't have to improvise, guess, or wonder if you're doing it right.

Every day has a clear purpose.

Every action has a reason.

**Every step is designed to accumulate progress.**

**This plan does not demand perfection.**

**It demands presence.**

**There will be easy days and uncomfortable days.**

**Days when you feel strong and days when you want to postpone.**

**That's normal.**

**The plan works despite that—not because everything is ideal.**

**You're not here to chase motivation.**

**You're here to build practical discipline.**

**It's not about doing everything.**

**It's about doing what's required today.**

**If one day isn't perfect, the process isn't canceled.**

**It continues.**

**If one day you fail, you don't move backward.**

**You resume.**

**If one day you doubt, you return to the plan.**

**This process was designed for real life—**

**with work, stress, responsibilities, and fatigue.**

**You don't need extra time.**

**You need order.**

**Before you begin, I want you to be clear on three simple rules:**

**1 Follow the days in order. Don't skip, don't jump ahead, don't mix.**

**2 Execute before you evaluate. Don't judge the process in the first few days.**

**3 Trust accumulation. Change isn't always visible right away, but it's always being built.**

**Throughout this plan, you will learn to:**

- make better decisions without fighting yourself
- listen to real signals from your body

- reduce mental noise around food and exercise
- create habits that sustain themselves

**There are no punishments.**

**No extremes.**

**No tricks.**

**There is structure, consistency, and coherence.**

**If you've made it this far, it's because you're ready.**

**Not to try one more time—**

**but to do it right.**

**Turn the page.**

**Day 1 isn't waiting for motivation.**

**It's waiting for action.**

# 4

# DAY 1 – STARTING POINT AND MEASUREMENT

Today, you are not going to change your body.
Today, you are going to put it in order.
And that is far more important than it seems.

Most people begin a weight-loss process without knowing exactly where they're starting from.

They don't measure.

They don't observe.

They don't record.

They just "start."

That mistake is what later creates doubt, anxiety, and abandonment—

days or weeks down the line:

*Am I making progress?*

*Is this working?*

*Should I change something?*

Today, we avoid all of that.

The purpose of Day 1

**Day 1 does not exist to demand anything from you.**
**It exists to establish a clear and honest baseline.**
**There is no judgment.**
**No guilt.**
**No comparison to anyone else.**
**Only data.**
**When you know exactly where you are,**
**every small improvement becomes visible.**
**And what's visible becomes motivating.**
**What to do today**
**1️⃣ Record your starting point**
**Take 15–20 minutes and record the following:**
• **Body weight**
*(If you have a scale, use it. If not, continue anyway.)*
• **Basic measurements**
*(Waist, hips, chest — you don't need to be perfect.)*
• **How you feel physically**
*(Energy, fatigue, digestion, sleep)*
• **How you feel mentally**
*(Stress, anxiety, motivation, clarity)*
**Write it down.**
**Don't keep it in your head.**
**This is not to punish yourself later.**
**It's to prove progress to yourself down the road.**
**2️⃣ Observe a full day without trying to change everything**
**Today, you are NOT making radical changes.**
**You are observing yourself:**
• What time do you eat?
• Do you eat from hunger or from habit?
• How often do you actually move?
• How much water do you drink?
• What time do you go to bed?

**Observation creates awareness.**

**And awareness is the first real change.**

**3️⃣ Make a simple commitment (not a heroic one)**

**Write or say out loud:**

*"For the next 30 days, I will follow this plan day by day, not seeking perfection—only consistency."*

**Don't promise results.**

**Promise execution.**

**What to avoid today**

- ❌ Don't start an extreme diet
- ❌ Don't punish yourself for what you see
- ❌ Don't try to "compensate"
- ❌ Don't compare yourself to anyone

**Today is not about winning.**

**It's about preparing the ground.**

**What to focus on**

- Honesty, not aesthetics
- Process, not results
- Clarity, not emotion

**This day may seem simple…**

**but it's what makes the rest of the plan work.**

**Before closing the day**

**Breathe and remember:**

- You're not starting from zero
- You're starting from the truth
- And that changes everything

**Tomorrow, we don't improvise.**

**Tomorrow, we begin activating the body.**

**Close this day calmly.**

**The process has already begun.**

# 5

# DAY 2 – FOUNDATIONS OF CHANGE

**Today, we're not chasing visible results.**
**Today, we're building the foundations that make results possible.**

The body doesn't change when it's forced all at once.

It changes when it receives clear, repeated signals that something is different.

Day 2 is about sending those first signals.

Not big sacrifices.

Not complicated rules.

Just basic order.

Today's goal

Establish three essential foundations:

1 Mindful eating

2 Basic movement

3 Hydration and rest

Nothing more. Nothing less.

When these three elements begin to align, the body responds faster than you imagine.

**What to do today**

**1️⃣ Eat with awareness, not anxiety**

Today you don't need to change everything you eat.

You need to change how you eat.

Apply these simple rules:

- Eat without rushing
- Chew more
- Stop when you're satisfied, not stuffed
- Avoid eating in front of screens when you can

Awareness reduces overeating effortlessly—

not because you restrict yourself, but because you listen.

**2️⃣ Move with intention**

Today is not a day for extreme workouts.

Do 20–30 minutes of basic movement, such as:

- walking
- mobility work
- stretching
- light activity that slightly elevates your heart rate

The message to your body is simple:

"We're moving again."

And that message matters more than intensity.

**3️⃣ Prioritize water and rest**

Many symptoms we confuse with hunger are dehydration or fatigue.

Today:

- Drink water regularly
- Try going to bed a little earlier
- Reduce stimulation before sleep

Better sleep makes every decision tomorrow easier.

**What to avoid today**

- ❌ Eating impulsively
- ❌ Training until exhaustion
- ❌ Skipping meals to "speed things up"
- ❌ Thinking this is too little

**Simple, done well, beats extreme, done inconsistently.**

**What to focus on**

- Rhythm, not speed
- Presence, not perfection
- Consistency, not heroic effort

**Today, your body begins to notice the change—**
**maybe not in the mirror...**
**but in your energy, digestion, or mental clarity.**
**That is real progress.**

**Before closing the day**

**Remind yourself:**

- You are building a system
- You are not improvising
- You are not fighting your body
- You are cooperating with it

**Tomorrow, we keep moving forward—step by step, without extremes.**

## 6

## DAY 3 – MOVEMENT AND ENERGY

Today, your body begins to understand that this is not just another attempt.

It begins to notice consistency.

Movement doesn't exist only to burn calories.

It exists to activate systems, improve mood, regulate appetite,

and remind the body that it's alive.

When you move well, everything else becomes easier.

Today's goal

Build a positive relationship with movement.

Not punishment.

Not obligation.

Movement as a tool—not a penance.

Today, we're looking for energy, not exhaustion.

What to do today

1️⃣ Move with intention (30 minutes)

Choose an activity you can sustain without hatred or suffering:

- brisk walking
- cycling

- a light at-home routine
- mobility work + basic exercises
- any activity that slightly elevates your heart rate

**Simple rule:**

**You should finish with more energy than you started with.**

**If you finish exhausted, it was too much.**

**2️⃣ Activate your body throughout the day**

**In addition to your main movement, add micro-movements:**

- stand up every hour
- walk for 5 minutes
- stretch
- take deep breaths

**These small stimuli keep your metabolism active without stress.**

**3️⃣ Observe how your body responds**

**Today, pay attention to:**

- your energy
- your mood
- your appetite
- your mental clarity

**Don't judge.**

**Just observe.**

**The body is always communicating.**

**Learning to listen is part of the process.**

**What to avoid today**

- ❌ Training out of guilt
- ❌ Thinking "if it doesn't hurt, it doesn't work"
- ❌ Comparing yourself to others
- ❌ Forcing paces you can't sustain

**The right movement adds—it doesn't take away.**

**What to focus on**

- Regularity, not intensity
- Sensations, not numbers
- Accumulated progress, not perfection

**Today, you're not training for an event.**

**You're training for a life that works.**

**Before closing the day**

**Remember this:**

- The body loves movement
- It hates punishment
- It responds best when it feels safe

**What you did today may seem simple.**

**But it's exactly what allows the process to move forward without friction.**

**Tomorrow, we'll work on something essential:**

**daily rhythm and consistency—**

**where most people fall off.**

# 7

# DAY 4 – DAILY RHYTHM AND CONSISTENCY

**The problem isn't starting.**
**The problem is continuing.**

Most people have the ability to do things right for a few days.

What they lack isn't strength—it's rhythm.

The body doesn't change through spikes of effort.

It changes through consistent signals.

Today, we establish that rhythm.

Today's goal

Create a realistic daily pattern you can repeat without friction.

Not the ideal rhythm.

Not the perfect rhythm.

The possible rhythm.

Because what can be repeated is sustained.

And what is sustained transforms.

What to do today

### 1️⃣ Define your baseline rhythm

**Answer honestly:**

- What time do you usually eat?
- What time can you move without stress?
- What time can you rest best?

**Don't adjust your life to the plan.**

**Adjust the plan to your life.**

**A system that doesn't fit your reality is destined to be abandoned.**

### 2️⃣ Establish anchor times

**Choose three daily anchor points:**

- one main meal
- one movement window
- one end-of-day closing moment

**They don't need to be exact to the minute.**

**Just consistent.**

**These anchors reduce decision fatigue and prevent improvisation.**

### 3️⃣ Do the same thing as yesterday (no more)

**Today, don't add anything new.**

**Repeat:**

- mindful eating
- basic movement
- hydration
- rest

**Repetition is what teaches the body this is serious.**

**What to avoid today**

- ❌ Changing the plan every day
- ❌ Pushing harder just because "you feel good"
- ❌ Thinking repetition is boring
- ❌ Skipping habits due to mental laziness

**Novelty motivates.**

**Repetition transforms.**

**What to focus on**

- Flow, not rigidity
- Making it easy, not making it hard
- Following through, not impressing

**Today, progress isn't visible.**

**It's being consolidated.**

**Before closing the day**

**Remind yourself:**

- The body learns through repetition
- The mind calms down with structure
- Consistency beats intensity

**If today you did the same thing as yesterday, you won.**

**Even if it feels like very little.**

**Tomorrow, we'll move into something essential:**

**water, rest, and recovery—three factors many people ignore**

**and then wonder why they stall.**

# 8

# DAY 5 – WATER, REST, AND RECOVERY

The invisible factors that determine whether you lose weight or not

Most people believe that losing weight depends only on what they eat

or how much they exercise.

That belief is incomplete... and dangerous.

Because even if you eat "well" and move every day,

if you don't rest and recover,

the body enters survival mode.

And a body in survival mode does not burn fat.

It protects it.

Today, we're going to work on the three factors almost no one takes seriously,

yet they determine the success or failure of the entire process:

water, rest, and recovery.

Today's goal

- **Optimize the body's internal environment**
- **Reduce physiological stress**
- **Make fat loss easier—without more effort**

**Today, we don't do more.**

**Today, we do better.**

**1️⃣ The real role of water in weight loss**

**Water is not generic advice.**

**It is a metabolic tool.**

**When the body is dehydrated:**

- energy drops
- hunger increases
- digestion slows down
- the body retains fluids
- metabolism becomes less efficient

**Many people think they're hungry...**

**when they're actually thirsty.**

**What to do with water today**

- Drink water regularly throughout the day
- Don't wait until you feel thirsty
- Prioritize plain water

**You don't need to obsess over exact liters.**

**You need consistency.**

**A simple reference:**

- one glass upon waking
- one before each meal
- one during movement
- one in the afternoon

**The body functions best when water is part of the day, not an isolated event.**

**2️⃣ Rest: the factor no one wants to hear about**

**Poor sleep sabotages any plan.**

**When you sleep too little or poorly:**

- hunger increases

- satiety decreases
- stress rises
- recovery drops
- the body becomes resistant to change

**This is not a lack of discipline.**

**It's physiology.**

**A tired body chooses what's easy—not what's right.**

**What to do with rest today**

**I'm not asking you to change your life.**

**I'm asking for a conscious adjustment:**

- go to bed a little earlier
- reduce screen time before sleep
- create a simple closing ritual

**Sleeping better is not a luxury.**

**It's a weight-loss strategy.**

**3 Recovery: the permission the body needs**

**Recovery is not laziness.**

**It is part of progress.**

**When you don't recover:**

- the body becomes inflamed
- appetite becomes erratic
- fatigue accumulates
- the process feels heavy

**Recovering allows the body to assimilate change.**

**What counts as recovery**

- rest
- stretching
- deep breathing
- moments of calm
- conscious pauses

**Not all progress comes from doing more.**

**Much of it comes from allowing the body to process.**

**What to avoid today**

- ❌ Living dehydrated
- ❌ Sleeping less "to make more progress"
- ❌ Ignoring signs of fatigue
- ❌ Thinking rest means falling behind

**The body does not move forward under threat.**

**It moves forward when it feels safe.**

**What to focus on**

- Creating a favorable internal environment
- Feeling better—not just looking different
- Making better decisions easier tomorrow

**Today, you're building the ground**

**where the body can change without resistance.**

**Before closing the day**

**Remind yourself:**

- The body does not burn fat when it's stressed
- It does not progress when it's exhausted
- It does not cooperate when it feels attacked

**But when it's well hydrated, well rested, and properly recovered...**

**it responds with surgical precision.**

**Tomorrow, we'll work on something just as important:**

**body awareness and your relationship with food—**

**where many people sabotage themselves without even realizing it.**

# 9

# DAY 6 – BODY AWARENESS AND HUNGER SIGNALS

Learning to listen to your body changes everything.

Most people don't eat because they're hungry.

They eat because it's time, because they're bored, because they're stressed,

or simply because food is available.

This day exists to break that disconnection.

When you can't tell the difference between real hunger and emotional hunger,

any plan becomes a constant struggle.

When you learn to listen to your body,

the process becomes much simpler.

Today's goal

- Restore communication with your body
- Reduce automatic impulses
- Eat with intention, not anxiety

Today is not about eating less.

It's about eating better informed.

**1️⃣ Real hunger vs. emotional hunger**

**Real hunger**

- Appears gradually
- Feels physical
- Is open to different foods
- Calms down after eating

**Emotional hunger**

- Appears suddenly
- Feels urgent
- Craves specific foods
- Is not easily satisfied

**Most overeating doesn't come from real hunger.**

**It comes from fatigue, stress, or habit.**

**Today, we observe this without judging ourselves.**

**2️⃣ Eating with presence**

**Eating while distracted confuses the body.**

**It doesn't register satiety.**

**It doesn't recognize limits.**

**Today, apply these simple rules:**

- Eat without screens whenever possible
- Chew more slowly
- Pause during meals
- Notice how you feel when you finish

**You don't need to count calories to control portions.**

**You need presence.**

**3️⃣ Satiety signals (that many people ignore)**

**The body signals fullness before being "full":**

- a sense of calm
- slower breathing
- less interest in food
- satisfaction, not heaviness

**Eating until you're stuffed is a learned habit.**

**Eating until you're satisfied is a skill that can be trained.**

**Today, we train that skill.**

**4️⃣ The role of stress in hunger**

**Stress distorts internal signals.**

**It increases cravings for fast, dense foods.**

**That's why:**

- sleeping better
- moving your body
- breathing
- taking pauses

**This is not a lack of control.**

**It's a biological response.**

**Reducing stress reduces uncontrolled hunger.**

**What to do today**

- Before eating, ask yourself:

*Is this physical hunger or emotional hunger?*

- Eat more slowly
- Stop before you're full
- Observe without blaming yourself

**What to avoid today**

- ❌ Eating on autopilot
- ❌ Skipping meals out of fear
- ❌ Punishing yourself for mistakes
- ❌ Believing control comes from restriction

**Real control comes from awareness.**

**What to focus on**

- Learning, not doing it perfectly
- Observing patterns
- Reconnecting with real signals

**Today may feel uncomfortable.**

**That's normal.**

**You're breaking automatic habits built over years.**

**Before closing the day**

**Remember this:**

- The body is always communicating
- The problem is that we stopped listening
- When you start listening again, the process becomes lighter

**Tomorrow, we'll close out Week 1 with something essential:**

**review, adjustments, and clarity—**

**so you can move forward without doubts.**

10

# DAY 7 – REVIEW AND ADJUSTMENTS

Progress is consolidated through evaluation, not improvisation.

You've reached the end of the first week.

And before moving forward, there's something you need to understand:

Real progress is not measured only by the mirror or the scale.

It's measured by what you're already doing differently.

Today is not about demanding more from yourself.

It's about building awareness, adjusting course, and continuing with clarity.

Most people fail because they never stop to review.

They either move forward blindly...

or they get frustrated because they "don't see changes."

Today, we do the opposite.

**Today's goal**

- **Evaluate without judging**
- **Adjust without punishing**
- **Reinforce what's already working**

**This day prevents future dropouts.**

**That's why it matters so much.**

**1️⃣ Review your week with honesty**

**Answer calmly:**

- Which habits did you follow consistently?
- What was easier than you expected?
- What felt more difficult?
- What changes did you notice in energy, hunger, or mood?

**Don't look for perfection.**

**Look for patterns.**

**A small change sustained**

**is worth more than a big change done sporadically.**

**2️⃣ Notice changes that aren't always visible**

**Many people quit because they're only looking for a number.**

**But the body often changes first in areas like:**

- reduced inflammation
- improved digestion
- greater mental clarity
- less anxiety
- better sleep

**If any of this has already improved, you're on the right path—**

**even if the scale hasn't moved much yet.**

**The body doesn't change everything at once.**

**It changes by systems.**

**3️⃣ Adjust without extremes**

**This is a day for fine-tuning, not revolutions.**

**Ask yourself:**

- Am I sleeping enough?
- Am I staying consistently hydrated?
- Am I eating with presence?
- Is my rhythm realistic?

**Adjust one thing—not everything.**

**Small changes are the ones that last.**

**4️⃣ Eliminate the "all-or-nothing" mindset**

**One imperfect day does not cancel the week.**

**One mistake does not invalidate the process.**

**The thought "I already failed"**

**is more damaging than any meal or bad day.**

**Here, we don't play all or nothing.**

**We play accumulated progress.**

**5️⃣ Reinforce commitment (not pressure)**

**Repeat your commitment—now with experience:**

*"I will continue this process day by day,*

*adjusting when necessary, without quitting."*

**Don't promise future results.**

**Promise continuity.**

**That's what changes everything.**

**What to avoid today**

- ❌ Comparing yourself to others
- ❌ Making impulsive decisions
- ❌ Changing the plan out of anxiety
- ❌ Punishing yourself for not being perfect

**This process is not built on guilt.**

**It's built on clarity.**

**What to focus on**

- What you're already doing well
- Maintaining your rhythm
- Trusting the process

**The first week is not meant to complete a physical transformation.**

**It's meant to create alignment.**

**And you're already achieving that.**

**Before closing the day**

**Breathe and acknowledge this:**

- You completed 7 days
- You didn't improvise
- You didn't quit
- You executed

**That alone already puts you ahead of over 90% of people who start.**

**Tomorrow, we enter Week 2 — Progress.**

**This is where the body begins to respond more clearly.**

**Not by magic.**

**By coherence.**

# 11

# DAY 8 – SMART ADJUSTMENTS

How to move forward without forcing the process

Reaching Day 8 is an important signal:
you're no longer starting—you're continuing.

And here's a truth many people ignore:

Not every day requires more effort.

Some days require better decisions.

This chapter exists to teach you how to adjust intelligently—

not how to apply pressure without purpose.

Today's goal

- Avoid early plateaus
- Fine-tune the system without breaking it
- Keep progress flowing

Today, we don't change everything.

Today, we optimize.

1️⃣ Why adjustments are necessary

The body is adaptable.

It learns quickly.

What creates change at the beginning
eventually becomes the new normal.

That's not a problem.

It's a sign of progress.

The mistake is responding to adaptation with extremes.

Today, we do the opposite.

2️⃣ Adjustment #1: Rhythm before intensity

If you feel good, don't speed up.

If you feel tired, don't punish yourself.

Check in on:

- Is your daily rhythm still realistic?
- Are you sleeping enough?
- Is your stress level manageable?

An overloaded body doesn't burn fat.

It holds onto it.

3️⃣ Adjustment #2: Quality over quantity

Many people believe that more exercise or less food
is always better.

It's not.

Sometimes the right adjustment is:

- eating more calmly
- moving better, not more
- sleeping better
- hydrating more consistently

The quality of the process defines the result.

4️⃣ Adjustment #3: Use body signals as your guide

Start using your body as a reference—
not just the plan.

Pay attention to:

- energy
- hunger

- digestion
- rest
- mood

**When something is off, the body lets you know.**

**Adjusting early prevents future frustration.**

**6️⃣ Adjustment #4: A continuity mindset**

**This is where many people sabotage themselves by thinking:**

*"I should be going faster."*

*"Maybe I need something more extreme."*

**That's anxiety—not intuition.**

**Remember:**

**real progress is quiet at first.**

**Today, we reaffirm commitment to the process—**

**not to urgency.**

**What to do today**

- Maintain your core habits
- Adjust only one thing if necessary
- Observe without judgment
- Continue

**What to avoid today**

- ❌ Changing everything at once
- ❌ Comparing yourself to others
- ❌ Increasing pressure out of anxiety
- ❌ Thinking slow progress equals failure

**Slow and steady progress is still progress.**

**What to focus on**

- Flow
- Sustainability
- Trust

**This day is invisible in the mirror...**

**but critical to the final result.**

**Before closing the day**

**Remember this:**

- Adjusting is not failing
- Adjusting is intelligence
- The body responds better when it feels heard

**Tomorrow, we'll move into something fundamental:**
**energy and body signals—**
**so you can keep moving forward with precision.**

12

# DAY 9 – ENERGY AND BODY SIGNALS

Learning to read your energy is learning to progress without getting stuck.

Energy is not just how you feel.

It's information.

The body is communicating all the time,

but most people don't know how to listen.

They ignore signals, force through them, or misinterpret them—

and then wonder why they feel exhausted, stuck, or give up.

This day exists for something fundamental:

Learning to read your energy as a guide, not as an obstacle.

Today's goal

- Recognize real energy patterns
- Differentiate normal fatigue from true exhaustion
- Use body signals to move forward with precision

**Today is not about doing more.**

**It's about doing better.**

**1️⃣ Energy is not constant (and it's not supposed to be)**

**One of the biggest mistakes is expecting to feel the same every day.**

**Energy:**

- rises
- falls
- adjusts
- responds to rest, stress, and rhythm

**That's normal.**

**The problem isn't having low-energy days.**

**The problem is interpreting them as failure.**

**Today, you learn not to sabotage yourself for feeling human.**

**2️⃣ Types of fatigue (not all mean you should stop)**

**Healthy fatigue**

- appears after movement
- improves with rest
- feels "clean"

**Accumulated fatigue**

- lingers
- affects mood
- creates irritability

**Exhaustion**

- consistently low motivation
- sleep problems
- intense cravings
- lack of mental clarity

**Each type requires a different response.**

**Forcing through exhaustion breaks the process.**

**Adjusting in time strengthens it.**

**3️⃣ How to use energy as a compass**

**Today, observe:**

- when you feel most energized
- which activities drain you
- which habits help you recover

**This isn't random.**

**It's valuable information.**

**When you align the plan with your energy peaks, everything becomes easier.**

**4 Move according to energy—not ego**

**Movement doesn't mean pushing yourself the same way every day.**

**High-energy days:**

- move with more intention
- take advantage of the momentum

**Low-energy days:**

- gentle movement
- walking
- mobility work
- recovery

**Both types of days count.**

**The mistake is believing only intense effort matters.**

**5 Hunger is also an energy signal**

**Intense hunger can signal:**

- lack of rest
- dehydration
- accumulated stress

**Food isn't always what the body is asking for.**

**Today, before eating, ask yourself:**

*What is my body really asking for right now?*

**That question changes decisions.**

**What to do today**

- Observe your energy throughout the day
- Adjust movement based on how you feel

- Prioritize rest if needed
- Follow the plan without forcing it

**What to avoid today**

- ❌ Ignoring real fatigue
- ❌ Forcing yourself out of guilt
- ❌ Thinking rest equals failure
- ❌ Comparing your energy to others

**Every body has its own rhythm.**

**What to focus on**

- Precision
- Listening
- Body respect

**Today, you're not trying to prove anything.**

**You're trying to align.**

**Before closing the day**

**Remember this:**

- Energy is a language
- The body is always communicating
- Those who learn to listen progress without fighting

**Tomorrow, we'll enter a key point:**

**progressing without anxiety—**

**so momentum doesn't turn into pressure.**

# 13

# DAY 10 – PROGRESS WITHOUT ANXIETY

How to move forward without pressure—and without quitting

Anxiety is one of the greatest enemies of physical change.

Not because it makes you weak,

but because it pushes you to make poor decisions.

Many people don't quit because the plan doesn't work.

They quit because they get desperate before it has time to work.

This day exists to teach you how to move forward

without rush, without pressure, and without self-sabotage.

Today's goal

- Reduce the urgency for immediate results
- Strengthen trust in the process
- Learn how to measure progress intelligently

**Today is not about speeding up.**

**It's about sustaining.**

### 1️⃣ Anxiety distorts how you perceive progress

**When you're anxious:**

- you exaggerate the negative
- you minimize the positive
- you doubt the process
- you want to change everything

**The problem isn't the plan.**

**It's the interpretation.**

**The body doesn't change in a straight line.**

**It changes in waves.**

**Days when it seems to move forward.**

**Days when it seems stuck.**

**Days when nothing makes sense.**

**All of that is normal.**

### 2️⃣ The mistake of measuring progress every day

**Weighing yourself daily, comparing yourself daily, or analyzing every detail fuels anxiety.**

**Weight fluctuates due to:**

- water
- digestion
- stress
- rest

**That does not mean regression.**

**Today, you begin to understand something essential:**

**Real progress is measured in trends—**

**not in isolated moments.**

### 3️⃣ Real signs of progress (beyond the scale)

**Start paying attention to:**

- increased energy
- reduced inflammation
- improved digestion

- greater mental clarity
- less anxiety around food

**These changes often appear before visible ones.**

**Ignoring them is a common mistake.**

**4️⃣ Patience as a strategy—not resignation**

**Being patient doesn't mean waiting passively.**

**It means executing without desperation.**

**Well-understood patience is an advanced form of discipline.**

**It's following the plan even when:**

- there's no applause
- there are no visible changes
- there's no immediate confirmation

**That's what separates those who achieve lasting results**

**from those who quit.**

**5️⃣ What to do when anxiety shows up**

**When you feel the urge to change something, do this:**

**1 Breathe**

**2 Check whether you followed today's plan**

**3 Remember that 10 days do not define a process**

**4 Continue**

**Never make important decisions from anxiety.**

**What to do today**

- Execute the day exactly as designed
- Avoid measuring everything
- Observe internal signals
- Trust

**What to avoid today**

- ❌ Changing the plan out of impatience
- ❌ Comparing yourself to others
- ❌ Thinking "it's not working"
- ❌ Looking for shortcuts

**Shortcuts create anxiety.**

**Systems create results.**

**What to focus on**

- Continuity
- Coherence
- Accumulation

**Today, progress doesn't shout.**

**It whispers.**

**And if you keep listening,**

**it will become undeniable.**

**Before closing the day**

**Remind yourself:**

- The body changes when it feels safe
- Urgency creates resistance
- Calm builds results

**Tomorrow, we'll work on something essential for many people:**

**real hunger vs. emotional hunger—**

**from an even more practical perspective.**

# 14

# DAY 11 – REAL HUNGER VS. EMOTIONAL HUNGER

Regaining control starts by knowing what your body is asking for.

Not everything that feels like hunger actually is.

And understanding this difference changes everything.

Many people believe they fail because they "lack control."

The truth is, they were never taught how to distinguish signals.

Today, you'll learn to clearly identify what your body is asking for

and what your emotions are asking for—

not to restrict yourself,

but to make better decisions.

Today's goal

• Identify patterns of real hunger and emotional hunger

- **Reduce automatic impulses**
- **Make conscious decisions without fighting yourself**

**Today is not about eating less.**

**It's about eating with clarity.**

**1️⃣ How real hunger shows up**

**Real hunger:**

- appears gradually
- is felt in the body (empty stomach, low energy)
- is open to different foods
- calms down after eating

**It's a physiological signal.**

**It's not urgent.**

**It's not desperate.**

**When you respond to real hunger with appropriate food,**

**the body regulates itself.**

**2️⃣ How emotional hunger shows up**

**Emotional hunger:**

- appears suddenly
- is felt in the mind
- craves specific foods
- often shows up with stress, fatigue, or boredom

**It's not asking for food.**

**It's asking for relief.**

**Eating from this place rarely brings real satisfaction.**

**That's why the cycle repeats.**

**3️⃣ The common mistake: fighting emotional hunger**

**Trying to "control" emotional hunger with willpower usually fails.**

**Not because you're weak,**

**but because it can't be solved with restriction.**

**Emotional hunger is better regulated through:**

- rest

- pauses
- movement
- breathing
- structure

Today, you learn to respond—not repress.

### 4 The conscious pause (a key tool)

When you feel the urge to eat, take a 60-second pause and ask:

- *Is this physical hunger or emotional hunger?*
- *What happened just before this feeling?*
- *What do I really need right now?*

Sometimes it will be food.

Sometimes it will be rest.

Sometimes it will be movement.

Sometimes it will be breathing.

Responding correctly prevents overeating without effort.

### 5 Eating without guilt changes your relationship with your body

Guilt intensifies emotional hunger.

When you eat with guilt:

- awareness drops
- eating speeds up
- you eat more than you need

When you eat with permission and presence,
the body regulates itself.

This process is not based on prohibition.

It's based on understanding.

What to do today

- Observe your signals before eating
- Take conscious pauses
- Respond with intention
- Eat without guilt

**What to avoid today**

- ✖ Eating on automatic impulse
- ✖ Judging yourself for feeling hunger
- ✖ Restricting out of fear
- ✖ Believing control comes from punishment

**Real control comes from clarity.**

**What to focus on**

- Learning patterns
- Reducing mental friction
- Improving your relationship with food

**Today, you're not "controlling" yourself.**

**You're training yourself.**

**Before closing the day**

**Remember this:**

- Hunger is a signal, not an enemy
- Understanding it sets you free
- Listening to your body reduces conflict

**Tomorrow, we'll work on something essential to consolidate progress:**

**practical discipline—the kind that doesn't depend on motivation.**

# 15

# DAY 12 – PRACTICAL DISCIPLINE

The discipline that works even when you don't feel like it

Most people believe discipline is willpower.

That it's about enduring.

That it's about pushing yourself.

That it's about doing things even when everything inside you wants to quit.

That idea is wrong.

And it's one of the main reasons so many people burn out, get frustrated, and give up.

Real discipline doesn't feel like a constant battle.

It feels like a system that supports you.

Today, you're going to understand what practical discipline really is—

and why it's the only kind that works long term.

Today's goal

- Redefine discipline
- Eliminate dependence on motivation

**• Build automatic, sustainable actions**

**Today, I won't ask more of you.**

**Today, I'll teach you how to rely less on effort.**

**1️⃣ The big lie about discipline**

**We were taught that discipline means doing hard things all the time.**

**That if it doesn't hurt, it doesn't work.**

**That if it's not difficult, it doesn't transform you.**

**That belief creates a huge problem:**

**People think that if one day they don't feel like it, they failed.**

**The truth is this:**

**Discipline is not about forcing yourself.**

**It's about making it easier to do the right thing.**

**2️⃣ Practical discipline vs. heroic discipline**

**Heroic discipline**

- depends on motivation
- demands constant force
- breaks down with fatigue
- is not sustainable

**Practical discipline**

- depends on structure
- reduces decisions
- adapts to good days and bad days
- holds up over time

**This book is built on practical discipline.**

**That's why the plan is daily.**

**That's why it's simple.**

**That's why it doesn't depend on feeling good.**

**3️⃣ The golden rule: keep it small, but do it every time**

**A common mistake is believing that more is always better.**

**In reality:**

- a small action done well
- repeated consistently

**beats any extreme effort done sporadically.**
**Today, we reaffirm this:**
**better incomplete than nonexistent.**
**A day where you did something**
**is better than a day where you did nothing.**

**4 How real discipline is built**

**Discipline is built when:**

- the environment supports you
- the plan is clear
- expectations are realistic
- progress is visible

**Not when you punish yourself.**
**That's why:**

- we don't improvise
- we don't change the plan based on emotion
- we don't demand perfection

**We execute.**
**We adjust.**
**We continue.**

**5 What to do when you don't feel like it**

**This is the key point.**
**When you don't feel like it:**

**1 Lower the target**
**2 Do the minimum version**
**3 Complete it**
**4 Continue**

**You don't need motivation to move for 10–20 minutes.**
**You don't need inspiration to eat mindfully.**
**You need structure—not emotion.**

**What to do today**

- Execute the day even if it's not perfect

- Do what's required, not what feels appealing
- Complete the minimum
- Continue

**What to avoid today**

- ✖ Waiting for motivation
- ✖ Forcing yourself out of guilt
- ✖ Thinking one low day invalidates everything
- ✖ Confusing discipline with punishment

**Real discipline protects the process.**

**What to focus on**

- Continuity
- Simplicity
- Trust

**Today, you're not proving strength.**

**You're building reliability with yourself.**

**Before closing the day**

**Remind yourself:**

- Discipline isn't harsh
- It's clear
- And when it's clear, it becomes natural

**Tomorrow, we'll move into something just as powerful:**

**continuity—the key that separates temporary results from real, lasting results.**

# 16

# DAY 13 – CONTINUITY

The quiet force that creates inevitable results

Most people don't fail because they don't know what to do.

They fail because they don't sustain what they already know.

Continuity isn't exciting.

It doesn't look good on social media.

It doesn't deliver instant dopamine.

But it is the most powerful force that exists
when it comes to transforming the body—
and life.

This chapter exists so you understand something few people truly grasp:

When continuity shows up,
results stop being a possibility
and become inevitable.

Today's goal

- **Turn actions into identity**
- **Eliminate the "starting over" mindset**
- **Understand why continuing matters more than any extreme effort**

**Today, we're not doing something new.**

**Today, we make sure what you're already doing stays.**

**1️⃣ The invisible mistake: living in cycles, not processes**

**Many people live like this:**

- they start
- they move forward
- they get tired
- they quit
- they blame themselves
- they start again

**That cycle is exhausting.**

**And it builds nothing.**

**Continuity breaks that pattern.**

**Continuing doesn't mean doing it perfectly.**

**It means not stopping the process.**

**2️⃣ Continuity is not repeated intensity**

**A common mistake is thinking continuity means doing the same intense thing every day.**

**It doesn't.**

**Continuity means:**

- adapting when you're tired
- reducing without quitting
- adjusting without breaking
- moving forward even on low days

**A process that only works on good days is not a process.**

**3️⃣ The body changes when it stops "expecting abandonment"**

Here is a deep truth:

The body responds better when it feels the change is real.

When you repeat habits for days and weeks,
the body stops resisting.
It stops "defending" the old state.
It starts cooperating.
Continuity builds physiological trust.
And when that happens,
change accelerates without force.

4️⃣ Continuity becomes identity

When you continue, something shifts inside you.
You stop saying:
*"I'm trying to lose weight."*
And you start living as:
*"I'm someone who takes care of myself."*
Continuity doesn't just change your body.
It changes who you believe you are.
And when identity changes,
maintaining results becomes natural.

5️⃣ What to do when continuity feels boring

This is crucial.
There will be days when everything feels flat.
When there's no emotion.
When there are no visible results.
That's where most people quit.
But that's also where results are locked in.
When there's no excitement
and you continue anyway,
you're building something that doesn't break.

What to do today

- Repeat the core habits
- Do it without chasing emotion

- Follow through even if it doesn't feel special
- Continue

**What to avoid today**

- ❌ Looking for new motivation
- ❌ Changing the plan out of boredom
- ❌ Believing it only works if it feels intense
- ❌ Stopping because "you already know this"

**Knowledge without continuity is worthless.**

**What to focus on**

- Identity
- Process
- Inevitability

**Today, you're crossing an invisible line.**
**From here on, quitting no longer makes sense—**
**because the system is working.**

**Before closing the day**

**Burn this into your mind:**

- Continuity beats talent
- Continuity beats motivation
- Continuity beats time

**When you continue long enough,**
**you win.**
**No rush.**
**No noise.**
**No drama.**
**Tomorrow, we'll move into a key moment:**
**the mid-point evaluation—**
**where many people panic...**
**and you'll learn to use it to your advantage.**

# 17

# DAY 14 – WEEKLY EVALUATION

How to measure without sabotaging yourself—and move forward with clarity

Reaching Day 14 is a critical point.

Not because of the number—

but because of what it represents.

This is where many people look at the mirror, the scale, or their body...

and make poor decisions.

They apply pressure.

They get frustrated.

They change everything.

Or they quit.

This chapter exists so you do the opposite.

Today's goal

- Evaluate without emotion
- Measure without anxiety
- Adjust without destroying the process

**Today, we're not looking to confirm perfection.**
**We're looking for the right direction.**

### 1️⃣ Evaluation is not judgment

**The word "evaluation" often triggers fear—**
**because many people use it to punish themselves.**
**Not here.**
**To evaluate is to observe data,**
**not to attack your identity.**
**A common mistake is thinking:**
*"If I don't see big changes, something is wrong."*
**That's false.**
**At two weeks, the body:**

- is still adapting
- is still regulating fluids
- is still learning the new rhythm

**Not all change is immediate or visible.**

### 2️⃣ What to actually evaluate on Day 14

**Today, review these areas honestly:**

**◆ Habits**

- Are you eating with more awareness?
- Are you moving more consistently?
- Are you sleeping better?

**◆ Energy**

- Is your energy more stable?
- Do you feel less heavy?

**◆ Relationship with food**

- Fewer impulses?
- More clarity while eating?

**These indicators often appear**
**before obvious physical change.**

### 3️⃣ The mistake of overvaluing the scale

**The scale shows one data point—**
**not the full truth.**

**Weight can fluctuate due to:**

- water
- digestion
- stress
- rest

**Using the scale as an absolute judge**
**is a mental trap.**
**Today, if you choose to weigh yourself,**
**do it with this rule in mind:**
**The scale informs—it does not define.**

**4️⃣ How to interpret results correctly**

**If progress is visible:**

- don't rush
- don't change anything
- continue

**If progress is minimal:**

- don't panic
- review habits
- adjust one thing
- continue

**If you see no change:**

- review sleep and stress
- review consistency
- maintain the plan
- continue

**The mistake isn't slow progress.**

**The mistake is abandoning a system that's already working.**

**5️⃣ Smart adjustments (not emotional ones)**

**Today, only this is allowed:**

- one small adjustment, if needed
- never drastic changes

**Examples of correct adjustments:**

- improving schedules
- sleeping better
- eating with more presence
- reducing stress

**Examples of incorrect adjustments:**

- eating less out of anxiety
- training more out of guilt
- changing everything "to speed things up"

**6️⃣ The trap of "I should be further along"**

**That phrase destroys processes.**
**There is no universal "should."**
**There is your process—**
**with your body, your history, and your rhythm.**
**Comparing yourself to unrealistic expectations**
**only creates friction.**
**And friction slows progress.**

**What to do today**

- Evaluate calmly
- Write down observations
- Adjust only if necessary
- Continue

**What to avoid today**

- ❌ Making decisions from emotion
- ❌ Comparing yourself to others
- ❌ Thinking you failed
- ❌ Changing the entire plan

**This day is not for impulsive action.**
**It's for fine-tuning the machine.**

**What to focus on**

- Direction, not speed
- Process, not perfection
- Consistency, not immediate results

**Today, you mark something important:**

**You are not someone who quits when it's time to evaluate.**

**You are someone who grows stronger by observing.**

**Before closing the day**

**Remind yourself:**

- Two weeks is progress
- Evaluation is maturity
- Continuing is power

**Tomorrow begins Week 3 — Transformation.**

**This is where the body starts responding more clearly.**

**Not because you forced it—**

**but because you sustained it.**

# 18

# DAY 15 – VISIBLE CHANGE

When the body begins to show what consistency has built

Reaching Day 15 is not a coincidence.

It's a consequence.

From this point on, many people begin to notice visible signals:

slightly looser clothes, less inflammation, a lighter feeling,

better posture, more energy.

And this is where something important happens:

The body starts to change...

and the mind can become the greatest risk.

This chapter exists to make sure that change is consolidated—

not sabotaged.

Today's goal

- Acknowledge change without euphoria
- Maintain coherence as results appear

- **Avoid classic "mid-process" mistakes**

**Today, we don't celebrate by rushing ahead.**

**Today, we secure the final result.**

**1️⃣ Visible change is an effect—not a goal**

**When you start seeing changes, it's easy to think:**

*"It worked. I can relax."*

*"I can speed things up."*

*"I can change the plan."*

**That mindset has destroyed more processes than any single meal or bad day ever could.**

**Visible change is not the finish line.**

**It's a signal that the system is working.**

**And when something works...**

**you don't modify it impulsively.**

**2️⃣ The kinds of changes that usually appear at this stage**

**Midway through the process, many people notice:**

- less inflammation
- a lighter waist or abdomen
- improved muscle tone
- more stable energy
- a healthier relationship with food

**These changes are usually cumulative, not dramatic.**

**And that's exactly what makes them sustainable.**

**3️⃣ The mistake of accelerating when things are going well**

**This is one of the most common errors:**

*"If this works, more must work even better."*

**So they:**

- eat less
- train more
- sleep worse
- demand more from themselves

**The result: fatigue, anxiety, and stagnation.**

**The body progresses best when it feels safe—**
**not when it's pressured.**

**4️⃣ Visible change is also internal**

**Beyond physical changes, check whether you're noticing:**

- more self-control
- less anxiety
- greater mental clarity
- stronger discipline
- increased confidence

**These changes are even more important than the physical ones.**

**Because when the mind changes,**
**the body maintains the result.**

**5️⃣ How to behave when results start showing**

**Clear rules at this stage of the process:**

- Don't change the plan
- Don't rush ahead
- Don't demand more
- Don't relax too much

**The correct formula is simple:**
**continue exactly as you are.**

**Continuity is what turns initial change**
**into real transformation.**

**What to do today**

- Follow the plan exactly as it is
- Observe changes calmly
- Reinforce core habits
- Maintain your rhythm

**What to avoid today**

- ❌ Celebrating by breaking the system
- ❌ Speeding up out of emotion

- ❌ Comparing yourself to others
- ❌ Thinking "it's already done"

**The body is still in a deep adjustment phase.**

**What to focus on**

- Coherence
- Stability
- Maintaining what already works

**Today, you're not looking for more.**

**You're looking for better.**

**Before closing the day**

**Burn this into your mind:**

- Visible change is a consequence
- Consistency is the cause
- If you maintain the cause, the effect continues

**Tomorrow, we'll enter a critical point:**

**hunger control—**

**when the body truly begins to regulate itself.**

# 19

# DAY 16 – HUNGER CONTROL

When the body stops fighting and starts cooperating

For many people, hunger has been the main enemy for years.

An uncomfortable, urgent, uncontrollable sensation that seems to sabotage every attempt at change.

But here's a truth that almost no one explains properly:

Hunger is not the problem.

Dysregulated hunger is.

Today, we begin to see something powerful:

when the body receives coherence, hunger organizes itself.

Today's goal

- Understand why hunger begins to stabilize
- Learn to trust the body's signals
- Avoid fear when appetite changes

Today, we don't fight hunger.

**Today, we learn how to use it to our advantage.**

**1 Why hunger begins to change at this stage**

**After more than two weeks of coherence:**

- better sleep
- better hydration
- regular movement
- lower stress
- consistent habits

**The body begins to feel safe.**

**And when the body feels safe:**

- impulses decrease
- appetite regulates
- satiety improves

**This isn't magic.**

**It's physiology working the way it's supposed to.**

**2 The mistake of getting scared when hunger decreases**

**This is a common form of self-sabotage:**

*"I'm not as hungry anymore...*

*am I eating too little?"*

**That fear leads many people to:**

- eat out of anxiety
- override internal signals
- distrust their own body

**Regulated hunger is not dangerous.**

**It's a sign of balance.**

**As long as you have energy, mental clarity, and good sleep,**

**your body is doing fine.**

**3 Regulated hunger vs. suppressed hunger**

**It's important to distinguish between the two:**

**Suppressed hunger**

- comes from restriction

- creates anxiety
- rebounds

**Regulated hunger**

- comes from coherence
- feels stable
- doesn't dominate decisions

**This process aims for the second.**
**It's not about forcing yourself to eat less.**
**It's about needing less—without suffering.**

**4️⃣ What to do when hunger shows up**

**Today, we use a simple rule:**
**Respect hunger—but don't hand it control.**
**If real hunger appears:**

- eat with awareness
- without guilt
- without rush

**If emotional hunger appears:**

- identify the emotion
- breathe
- move
- decide

**Control doesn't come from ignoring hunger.**
**It comes from understanding it.**

**5️⃣ The fear of "losing control" is the final obstacle**

**Many people have lived in extremes for so long**
**that when the body regulates itself, they don't trust it.**
**They believe that if they stop monitoring everything,**
**everything will spiral out of control.**
**The truth is this:**
**When the system works,**
**control no longer depends on constant vigilance.**
**It depends on habits.**
**And those habits are already being built.**

**What to do today**

- Eat calmly
- Trust the signals
- Avoid eating out of fear
- Stay with the plan

**What to avoid today**

- ❌ Forcing yourself to eat without hunger
- ❌ Skipping meals out of fear
- ❌ Micromanaging every detail out of anxiety
- ❌ Believing control equals rigidity

**Real control is balance.**

**What to focus on**

- Body trust
- Stability
- Coherence

**Today, you're experiencing something many people never reach:**

**your body is beginning to cooperate with you.**

**Before closing the day**

**Remember this:**

- Regulated hunger is freedom
- The body knows how to self-regulate
- Your job is not to interfere with panic

**Tomorrow, we'll move into something powerful:**

**habit automation—**

**when the process begins to feel natural.**

20

# DAY 17 – METABOLISM AND MOVEMENT

**When your body starts working in your favor**

For years, you were told that metabolism was something that could be "damaged,"

that it could "shut down," or that it depended solely on age or genetics.

That created fear, frustration, and resignation.

The truth is much simpler—

and much more powerful:

Your metabolism is not broken.

It's responding to the context you gave it.

And when that context changes consistently,

metabolism responds.

Today, you'll understand how it actually works—

and how the right kind of movement activates it

without destroying you.

Today's goal

- **Understand what metabolism really is**
- **Use movement as an activator—not a punishment**
- **Facilitate fat burning without stress**

**Today, we're not chasing exhaustion.**

**We're aiming for efficiency.**

### 1️⃣ What metabolism really is (without the myths)

**Metabolism is not one thing.**

**It's a set of processes that determine how the body:**

- uses energy
- stores energy
- recovers
- adapts

**An efficient metabolism:**

- doesn't rely on extremes
- responds to consistent signals
- functions best with balanced rest and movement

**It's not "sped up" through suffering.**

**It's optimized through coherence.**

### 2️⃣ Why movement matters more than extreme exercise

**The body wasn't designed for isolated sessions of punishment.**

**It was designed to move regularly.**

**Movement:**

- improves metabolic sensitivity
- regulates appetite
- boosts energy
- facilitates fat utilization

**And here's something critical:**

**Moving more throughout the day**
**is often more effective**
**than training extremely hard once.**

**This book isn't about exhausted athletes.**

**It's about functional, sustainable bodies.**

**3️⃣ The mistake of "burn more to lose more"**

**This belief has destroyed thousands of processes.**

**Thinking:**

*"If I move more, I'll lose weight faster."*

**Usually leads to:**

- fatigue
- uncontrolled hunger
- stress
- stagnation

**The body burns fat when it feels safe—**

**not when it feels hunted.**

**4️⃣ Smart movement = cooperative metabolism**

**From this point on, movement serves three clear functions:**

1 **Activate** (walking, moving, changing posture)

2 **Stimulate** (simple routines, basic exercises)

3 **Recover** (mobility, stretching, breathing)

**When these three coexist,**

**metabolism optimizes itself without conflict.**

**5️⃣ How to use movement based on your energy**

**This is an advanced principle:**

- High-energy days → more intentional movement
- Low-energy days → gentle movement
- High-stress days → walking and breathing

**Every day counts.**

**The mistake is believing only intense days matter.**

**6️⃣ Stable metabolism vs. stressed metabolism**

**A stressed metabolism:**

- holds onto fat
- increases hunger

- lowers energy

**A stable metabolism:**

- uses energy efficiently
- regulates appetite
- adapts smoothly

**The difference isn't genetic.**

**It's contextual.**

**And today, you're building the right context.**

**What to do today**

- Move with intention
- Prioritize regularity over intensity
- Walk more
- Avoid prolonged sedentary periods

**What to avoid today**

- ✖ Training out of guilt
- ✖ Chasing exhaustion
- ✖ Forcing when the body asks for adjustment
- ✖ Believing more is always better

**Metabolism responds to clear signals—**

**not punishment.**

**What to focus on**

- Efficiency
- Flow
- Body cooperation

**Today, your body begins working with you—**

**not against you.**

**Before closing the day**

**Burn this in:**

- Metabolism adapts
- Movement guides it
- Coherence optimizes it

**When you understand this,**

**the process stops being a fight**
**and becomes an automatic system.**
**Tomorrow, we'll move into a decisive point:**
**habit automation—**
**when everything starts to feel natural.**

# 21

# DAY 18 – HABIT AUTOMATION

When you no longer have to push yourself to move forward

Real power isn't found in doing something once.

It's not even found in doing it for 30 days.

Real power is found in doing it without thinking.

When habits become automated:

- there's no struggle
- there's no negotiation
- there's no mental exhaustion

The body and mind simply function.

This chapter marks a point of no return.

Today's goal

- Understand how real habits are formed
- Stop depending on conscious effort
- Turn actions into automatic behavior

Today, we don't add anything new.

Today, we solidify what already exists.

**1️⃣ Why most people never automate habits**

**Most people fail because they:**

- change too quickly
- demand perfection
- break repetition
- quit once they "understand"

**Habits are not formed by understanding them.**

**They're formed by repetition—without drama.**

**And you've already been repeating for more than two weeks.**

**That matters.**

**2️⃣ How the body knows something is "real"**

**The body doesn't believe intentions.**

**It believes patterns.**

**When you do something:**

- on the same days
- in a similar way
- without long interruptions

**the body assumes:**

*"This is part of life now."*

**And it stops resisting.**

**That is automation.**

**3️⃣ The exact moment where many people self-sabotage**

**A dangerous thought appears here:**

*"I already understand this. I can relax."*

**And then they:**

- stop tracking
- improvise
- break schedules
- lose rhythm

**Not because they're weak—**

**but because they confuse understanding with integration.**

**Knowing something doesn't mean it already lives in you.**

**4️⃣ Signs your habits are already becoming automatic**

**Notice if you're experiencing this:**

- you eat more calmly without thinking about it
- you move without having to force yourself
- you choose better without debating
- it feels strange when you don't follow through

**That's the system taking over.**

**Don't interrupt it.**

**5️⃣ Automation is not rigidity—it's flow**

**Automating habits doesn't mean becoming rigid.**

**It means reducing friction.**

**When something is automatic:**

- it doesn't drain you
- it doesn't stress you
- it doesn't require motivation

**Rigidity breaks habits.**

**Flow sustains them.**

**6️⃣ The mistake of "waiting until it feels natural"**

**Many people say:**

*"Once it feels natural, I'll keep doing it."*

**The truth is the opposite:**

**It feels natural because you kept doing it.**

**Naturalness is the result—not the starting point.**

**What to do today**

- Repeat exactly what's already working
- Don't innovate
- Don't complicate
- Don't speed up

**Today, repetition is the win.**

**What to avoid today**

- ❌ Changing things out of boredom
- ❌ Thinking it's already "mastered"
- ❌ Trying new things out of anxiety
- ❌ Breaking the rhythm

**Simple actions repeated**

**beat brilliant ideas improvised.**

**What to focus on**

- Repetition
- Stability
- Quiet continuity

**Today doesn't feel epic.**

**But this is what builds results that last.**

**Before closing the day**

**Burn this in:**

- Automatic habits create freedom
- Freedom reduces effort
- Less effort equals more consistency

**From here on,**

**the process begins to move on its own.**

**Tomorrow, we'll enter something powerful:**

**a progress mindset—**

**when change is no longer negotiated.**

22

# DAY 19 – PROGRESS MINDSET

Thinking like the person who always moves forward—
even when they stumble

The difference between those who achieve lasting results and those who don't

isn't in the body.

It's in how they interpret what happens during the process.

Two people can do the exact same thing.

One progresses.

The other quits.

The difference is the progress mindset.

This chapter exists to install it.

Today's goal

• Eliminate the failure mindset

• Learn to interpret mistakes as information

• Solidify a way of thinking that doesn't move backward

**Today, we don't train the body.**

**Today, we armor the mind.**

**1️⃣ The "all-or-nothing" mindset destroys processes**

**Many people live by this logic:**

- If I do it perfectly, I continue
- If I fail, I quit

**That mindset doesn't allow real progress.**

**It only allows short streaks.**

**True progress is built through well-managed imperfections.**

**One bad day doesn't break a process.**

**What breaks it is how you interpret that day.**

**2️⃣ Progress is not the absence of mistakes**

**Here's an uncomfortable truth:**

**People who achieve real change also fail.**

**The difference is that they:**

- don't dramatize
- don't punish themselves
- don't restart from zero

**They adjust.**

**They continue.**

**They move forward.**

**A progress mindset doesn't eliminate mistakes.**

**It eliminates quitting.**

**3️⃣ Mistakes as data—not identity**

**Many people say:**

*"I failed."*

**But what actually happened was:**

*"One day didn't go as expected."*

**Confusing an event with identity destroys momentum.**

**Today, we install this rule:**

**A mistake is information—not a verdict.**

**And information, when used correctly, improves the system.**

### 4️⃣ How a person with a progress mindset thinks

**After a setback, they ask:**

- What happened?
- What can I adjust?
- How do I continue tomorrow?

**They don't think:**

- "I ruined everything"
- "I'm not good at this"
- "I'll start again on Monday"

**A progress mindset doesn't stop to punish itself.**

### 5️⃣ The power of continuing without drama

**This is one of the most powerful skills that exists:**

**Continuing without creating an emotional story.**

**No explanations.**

**No justifications.**

**No punishment.**

**You simply continue.**

**That builds an internal trust no one can take away from you.**

### 6️⃣ When identity begins to shift

**If you've made it this far, something has already changed.**

**You're starting to see yourself as:**

- someone who doesn't quit
- someone who adjusts
- someone who keeps going

**And when identity changes, results stop being fragile.**

**The body adapts to the dominant identity.**

**What to do today**

- Observe your thoughts
- Identify unnecessary dramatization

- Replace it with adjustment
- Continue

**What to avoid today**

- ❌ Thinking in absolutes
- ❌ Labeling yourself based on a mistake
- ❌ Restarting from zero
- ❌ Chasing perfection

**Perfection doesn't build progress.**

**Imperfect continuity does.**

**What to focus on**

- Learning
- Adjusting
- Moving forward

**Today, you're no longer the person who "tries."**

**You're the person who progresses.**

**Before closing the day**

**Burn this in:**

- Progress doesn't break
- It only pauses if you decide it does
- Continuing is power

**Tomorrow, we'll move into something deeply powerful:**

**body trust—**

**when body and mind fully align.**

# 23

# DAY 20 – BODY TRUST

When you stop doubting your body and start living in it

A lack of body trust doesn't come from the body.

It comes from years of failed attempts, broken promises, and constant struggle.

Many people don't hate their body.

They distrust it.

They don't believe it will respond.

They don't believe it will change.

They don't believe it can sustain results.

This day exists to change that.

Because when you rebuild trust in your body,

the process stops feeling fragile…

and becomes solid.

Today's goal

- Rebuild your relationship with your body
- Stop seeing it as a problem
- Start trusting its ability to adapt

**Today, we're not looking for external validation.**

**We're building internal trust.**

**1️⃣ Why body distrust sabotages results**

**When you don't trust your body:**

- you doubt your signals
- you over-monitor yourself
- you restrict out of fear
- you demand more than necessary

**That state creates tension.**

**And tension slows progress.**

**The body changes best when it feels safe—**

**not controlled.**

**2️⃣ Trust is not carelessness**

**This is an important distinction.**

**Trusting your body does not mean:**

- eating without awareness
- abandoning structure
- "doing whatever you want"

**Trust means:**

- listening to real signals
- responding with coherence
- maintaining habits without fear

**When understood correctly, trust strengthens discipline—**

**it doesn't weaken it.**

**3️⃣ Signs that trust is returning**

**Notice if you're starting to experience:**

- less anxiety around food
- less fear of "ruining it"
- more calm when making decisions
- greater connection to real sensations

**These are signs your internal system is aligning.**

**That is huge.**

**4 The body learns to trust when you keep going**

**Trust isn't built through promises.**

**It's built through repeated experience.**

**Every day you:**

- follow through
- adjust without quitting
- continue without punishing yourself

**you're proving to your body that this process is not an attack.**

**And when the body stops defending itself,**

**it cooperates.**

**5 The mistake of monitoring yourself all the time**

**Tracking every meal, every movement, every sensation...**

**isn't discipline.**

**It's fear.**

**And fear creates rigidity.**

**Today, we begin to loosen that extreme vigilance—**

**without losing structure.**

**Trust reduces friction.**

**And less friction equals more consistency.**

**6 When the body stops being the enemy**

**This is where something shifts deeply.**

**You stop thinking:**

*"My body always sabotages me."*

**And you start living as:**

*"My body responds when I'm consistent."*

**That belief changes everything.**

**What to do today**

- Eat calmly
- Listen to real signals
- Respond without fear
- Maintain structure

**What to avoid today**

- ❌ Over-monitoring out of anxiety
- ❌ Doubting every decision
- ❌ Controlling yourself out of fear
- ❌ Punishing yourself for imperfections

**Trust breaks through punishment.**

**It's built through coherence.**

**What to focus on**

- Calm
- Connection
- Stability

**Today, you don't need to prove anything.**

**You need to live in your body with respect.**

**Before closing the day**

**Burn this in:**

- Your body is not the problem
- It reflects your coherence
- When you trust, it responds

**Tomorrow, we'll enter a critical point:**

**a deep review of the process—**

**where we fine-tune the final stretch.**

# 24

# DAY 21 – TRANSFORMATION REVIEW

Pausing to recognize who you're becoming

Today is not just another day.

Today is a turning point.

Not because the process is ending—

but because you are no longer the same person who started.

Reaching Day 21 means something very important:

Change stopped being an attempt

and became a reality in motion.

This chapter exists so you recognize it, understand it, and secure it.

Today's goal

• Review the full transformation—not just the scale

• Identify what has already changed in an irreversible way

• Make sure what you've built doesn't get lost in the final stretch

**Today, we don't speed up.**

**Today, we reinforce.**

**1️⃣ Transformation doesn't happen only in the body**

**If you measure progress only by the mirror or the scale,**

**you're missing the most important part.**

**By this point, it's very likely you've already changed in areas like:**

- your relationship with food
- your ability to continue without drama
- the way you interpret mistakes
- your level of body awareness
- your daily discipline

**These changes are the real transformation.**

**The body follows the mind. Always.**

**2️⃣ Who you're no longer becoming (even if you don't notice)**

**Do this exercise honestly.**

**You're no longer:**

- the person who quits after the first mistake
- the person who lives in extremes
- the person who starts with excitement and disappears
- the person who fights their body

**It may not feel "epic."**

**But it's real.**

**And what's real is what lasts.**

**3️⃣ The dangerous Day 21 mistake: relaxing too much**

**A quiet thought often appears here:**

*"I already did it. I get it now. I can loosen up."*

**That thought has destroyed more processes**

**than any meal or bad day ever could.**

**Not because resting is bad—**

**but because it confuses understanding with consolidation.**

**Knowing something doesn't mean it's fully integrated.**

**Today, we don't loosen up.**

**Today, we secure it.**

**4️⃣ Deep review: the five key questions**

**Answer these calmly:**

1 What habits feel more natural today than they used to?

2 What decisions do you now make without debating so much?

3 Where do you feel less anxiety than at the beginning?

4 What did you do even on difficult days?

5 What do you never want to lose again?

**Your answers reveal who you're becoming.**

**5️⃣ Your body now knows this is real**

**After 21 days of coherence:**

- the body stops resisting
- metabolism cooperates
- appetite regulates more easily
- energy becomes more stable

**Not because you forced it—**

**because you sustained it.**

**This is the point where the body starts to say:**

*"This isn't temporary."*

**And when that happens, change becomes easier.**

**6️⃣ The difference between a result and a transformation**

**A result is something you can lose.**

**A transformation is something you carry with you.**

**If you went backward today (and you won't),**

**you couldn't do it the same way—**

**because you know too much, feel differently,**

**and you're more aware.**

**That is transformation.**

**What to do today**

- Review your entire process
- Recognize invisible progress
- Reinforce core habits
- Maintain your rhythm

**What to avoid today**

- ❌ Minimizing what you've achieved
- ❌ Comparing yourself to others
- ❌ Relaxing out of overconfidence
- ❌ Thinking "it's over"

**This isn't over.**

**It's consolidated.**

**What to focus on**

- Identity
- Stability
- Conscious continuity

**Today, you don't celebrate by breaking the system.**

**You celebrate by sustaining it.**

**Before closing the day**

**Burn this in deeply:**

- You've already changed
- The process works
- What comes next is final consolidation

**Tomorrow, we enter Week 4 — Consolidation.**

**This is where the result becomes rebound-proof.**

**Don't loosen up.**

**Don't rush.**

**Continue.**

# 25

# DAY 22 – MAINTAINING THE RHYTHM

The art of not sabotaging what's already working

Making it this far means something very clear: the process is working.

And precisely because of that,

this point can be dangerous.

Not because it's difficult—

but because of a false sense of safety.

Most people don't lose progress because of major mistakes.

They lose it because they loosen up when they shouldn't.

This chapter exists to make sure that doesn't happen to you.

Today's goal

- Maintain coherence without rigidity
- Avoid overconfidence
- Sustain the right rhythm through the finish line

**Today, we don't push.**

**Today, we protect.**

**1️⃣ The silent mistake: confusing comfort with permission**

**When the process starts to feel natural,**

**a subtle thought appears:**

*"I've got this under control."*

**And little by little:**

- you improvise more
- you neglect rest
- key habits loosen
- rhythm breaks

**Not all at once—**

**almost invisibly.**

**This mistake doesn't feel like sabotage...**

**it feels like "normal life."**

**But it breaks results.**

**2️⃣ Maintaining the rhythm is not about doing more**

**Here's an important truth:**

**Maintaining the rhythm does not mean increasing demands.**

**It means:**

- repeating what already works
- protecting key schedules
- respecting body signals
- not altering the system based on emotion

**The right rhythm is the one you can sustain without friction.**

**3️⃣ The body responds better to stability than to surprises**

**The body thrives on predictability.**

**When you:**

- eat consistently

- move regularly
- sleep better
- reduce stress

**the body cooperates.**

**When you start surprising it with unnecessary changes,**

**it responds with resistance.**

**Today, we reaffirm stability.**

**4️⃣ The "final push" trap**

**Some people think:**

*"I'm almost done—I'll give it one last push."*

**And then they:**

- train more
- eat less
- sleep worse

**That doesn't speed results up.**

**It complicates them.**

**The body doesn't need a final push.**

**It needs continuity without drama.**

**5️⃣ Maintaining rhythm is a high-level skill**

**Anyone can start with intensity.**

**Very few know how to maintain.**

**Maintain:**

- when it's no longer new
- when it's no longer exciting
- when urgency is gone

**That is mastery.**

**And this skill doesn't just change your body—**

**it changes your life.**

**6️⃣ Signs you're maintaining the rhythm well**

**Notice if you're experiencing:**

- less anxiety about "doing more"
- more calm in repetition

- more automatic decisions
- less mental exhaustion

**These are signs the system is well calibrated.**

**Don't disrupt it.**

**What to do today**

- Repeat the core habits
- Protect key schedules
- Prioritize rest
- Maintain the plan

**What to avoid today**

- ❌ Improvising out of confidence
- ❌ Increasing demands without reason
- ❌ Relaxing too much
- ❌ Thinking "it no longer matters"

**Every day still matters—**

**precisely because it's working.**

**What to focus on**

- Stability
- Process protection
- Conscious continuity

**Today, you're not trying to move faster.**

**You're making sure you don't move backward without noticing.**

**Before closing the day**

**Burn this in:**

- Progress is lost through small neglect
- Stability protects it
- Maintaining rhythm is intelligence

**Tomorrow, we enter a critical point:**

**rebound prevention—**

**where we seal the result.**

# 26

# DAY 23 – PREVENTING REBOUND

How to make sure the weight you lose never comes back

Fear of rebound isn't irrational.

It's experience.

Many people have lost weight before...

only to watch it return weeks or months later.

That creates frustration, distrust, and a dangerous feeling:

*"It always ends up the same."*

This chapter exists to break that pattern at the root.

Because rebound isn't inevitable.

It's the result of specific mistakes—

and today you're going to learn how to avoid them.

Today's goal

- Understand why rebound happens
- Eliminate the behaviors that cause it
- Make your results long-term proof

Today, we're not trying to lose more.

Today, we protect what you've earned.

1️⃣ Rebound doesn't happen in the body—it happens in the system

Here's the truth almost no one explains well:

The body doesn't "rebound" for no reason.

It rebounds when the system that supported it disappears.

Extreme diets work while they exist.

When they end, the body returns to the environment it knows.

This book is different because it isn't built on a temporary phase.

It's built on habits that continue.

2️⃣ The most common mistake: returning to your old life

After seeing results, many people think:

*"I can go back to how I used to live."*

And that's where rebound begins.

Not because one meal ruins everything—

but because the entire context shifts.

The body doesn't respond to isolated events.

It responds to patterns.

Let this be clear today:

You don't go backward. You adjust forward.

3️⃣ Emotional rebound (the most dangerous kind)

Rebound doesn't always start physically.

Sometimes it begins in the mind.

It shows up as:

- neglect
- "I'll get back on track tomorrow"
- constant improvisation
- loss of awareness

When the mind loosens too much, the body follows.

**This chapter prevents that quiet rebound.**

**4️⃣ The golden rule for preventing rebound**

**Keep this as law:**

**Never eliminate all your habits at the same time.**

**If you slip on one thing:**

- keep the rest
- adjust
- continue

**Rebound happens when everything breaks at once.**

**5️⃣ The role of sleep and stress in rebound**

**Many rebounds don't come from food.**

**They come from:**

- poor sleep
- chronic stress
- exhaustion

**A depleted body seeks survival—**

**and that often shows up as hunger, cravings, and loss of control.**

**Protecting your sleep protects your results.**

**6️⃣ How to think so you don't rebound**

**The right mindset is this:**

- I didn't "finish a plan"
- I'm living differently now

**When you see this as a phase that ends,**

**the body expects you to go back.**

**When you see it as a system that adapts,**

**the body stays with you.**

**What to do today**

- Reinforce the core habits
- Protect sleep
- Maintain structure
- Avoid extremes

**What to avoid today**

- ❌ Thinking "it's over"
- ❌ Returning to old patterns
- ❌ Breaking everything because of one mistake
- ❌ Punishing yourself for imperfections

**Rebound isn't prevented with fear.**

**It's prevented with continuous structure.**

**What to focus on**

- Stability
- Coherence
- The long term

**Today, you're not protecting a number.**

**You're protecting your new normal.**

**Before closing the day**

**Burn this in deeply:**

- Rebound is not destiny
- It's a consequence
- And you already know how to prevent it

**Tomorrow, we'll move into something essential:**

**smart flexibility—**

**so you can live without fear and without rigidity.**

27

# DAY 24 – SMART FLEXIBILITY

How to live without fear, without rigidity, and without losing results

One of the biggest mistakes in transformation processes

is confusing discipline with rigidity.

Believing that to maintain results you must live controlling yourself,

restricting yourself, or constantly saying "no."

That approach is not sustainable.

And sooner or later, it leads to rebound.

This chapter exists to teach you something essential:

Flexibility doesn't destroy results.

A lack of structure does.

When flexibility is intelligent,

it protects the process.

Today's goal

• Eliminate the fear of "going off plan"

- **Learn to be flexible without self-sabotage**
- **Integrate the process into real life**

**Today, we don't break the system.**

**Today, we make it livable.**

### 1️⃣ Extreme rigidity: the fastest path to quitting

**Rigidity looks like this:**

- constant fear of making mistakes
- guilt over any deviation
- anxiety about controlling everything
- feeling trapped

**That state cannot be sustained.**

**The body and mind eventually try to escape rigidity.**

**And when they do, they do it through excess.**

### 2️⃣ Smart flexibility vs. chaotic flexibility

**It's important to distinguish between the two.**

**Chaotic flexibility:**

- improvising without awareness
- breaking habits emotionally
- using "flexibility" as an excuse

**Smart flexibility:**

- choosing consciously
- maintaining core habits
- returning to rhythm without drama

**The key is not never deviating.**

**The key is knowing how to return quickly.**

### 3️⃣ The 80/20 rule applied to the body

**Here's a powerful principle:**

**Do things right 80% of the time,**

**and the remaining 20% takes care of itself.**

**When your core habits are solid:**

- one different meal doesn't ruin anything
- one different day doesn't break the process
- social life is not the enemy

**The mistake is living in the 20%—**
**or punishing yourself for it.**

**4 How to use flexibility without losing control**

**Before choosing something different, ask yourself:**

- Is this a conscious choice or an emotional reaction?
- Can I enjoy this without guilt?
- Can I return to rhythm tomorrow without drama?

**If the answer is yes, go ahead.**
**If not, it's not flexibility.**
**It's avoidance.**

**5 The body responds better when fear is removed**

**Fear creates tension.**
**Tension creates resistance.**
**Resistance slows progress.**
**When you eat, move, and live without constant fear,**
**the body cooperates more easily.**
**Well-used flexibility reduces stress—**
**and less stress equals better regulation.**

**6 Flexibility doesn't mean losing identity**

**Being flexible doesn't mean becoming who you used to be.**

**It means:**

- choosing from your new identity
- acting with awareness
- maintaining the system

**Your identity has already changed.**
**Flexibility is now built from that place.**

**What to do today**

- Allow yourself to choose consciously
- Maintain core habits
- Enjoy without guilt
- Return to rhythm

**What to avoid today**

- ❌ Living in fear of mistakes
- ❌ Punishing yourself for flexibility
- ❌ Using flexibility as an excuse
- ❌ Breaking everything because of one event

**Correct flexibility protects results.**

**What to focus on**

- Balance
- Conscious enjoyment
- Long-term stability

**Today, you're learning how to live well without losing yourself.**

**Before closing the day**

**Burn this in deeply:**

- You don't need rigidity to maintain results
- You need awareness
- Smart flexibility is freedom

**Tomorrow, we'll enter something crucial:**

**an active lifestyle—**

**where movement becomes part of life without effort.**

# 28

# DAY 25 – ACTIVE LIFESTYLE

**When movement stops being an obligation and becomes natural**

For years, many people were taught that exercise is something you either "do" or don't do—

an activity separate from life, locked into rigid schedules or extreme sessions.

That approach is one of the main reasons so many processes fail.

**The truth is this:**

**The body was not designed to train once in a while.**

**It was designed to move every day.**

This chapter exists to integrate movement into your life—

not to impose it on top of it.

**Today's goal**

- **Stop seeing movement as punishment**
- **Integrate physical activity naturally**

- **Build an active body without constant mental effort**

**Today, we're not talking about routines.**

**We're talking about how you live.**

**1️⃣ Movement vs. exercise (the difference that changes everything)**

**Exercise:**

- often feels like an obligation
- requires motivation
- is easy to abandon

**Movement:**

- is part of the day
- requires no negotiation
- sustains itself

**People who stay fit don't necessarily "train more."**

**They move more.**

And that changes everything.

**2️⃣ The body responds better to distributed movement**

Moving a little many times throughout the day
is often more effective than moving a lot once.

Simple examples:

- walking after meals
- taking the stairs
- moving every hour
- stretching
- changing positions

These actions:

- improve body sensitivity
- regulate appetite
- keep metabolism active
- reduce stiffness and stress

And they don't cause exhaustion.

**3️⃣ The mistake of waiting to "feel like it"**

Waiting for motivation to move is a trap.

**The desire comes after the movement—not before it.**

Today, we reinforce this principle:

**Move first.**

**Feel better later.**

Not the other way around.

### 4️⃣ Integrating movement into real life

An active lifestyle is built through small decisions:

- walking more
- sitting less
- moving between tasks
- choosing activities that involve movement

You don't need to change your life.

You need to activate your day.

### 5️⃣ Movement as an emotional regulator

Movement doesn't just change the body.

It changes your mental state.

Moving:

- reduces anxiety
- improves mood
- clears the mind
- regulates appetite

That's why, many times, when you move more...

you eat better without even thinking about it.

### 6️⃣ An active body ages differently

A body that moves:

- recovers better
- maintains strength
- preserves mobility
- adapts more easily

This process isn't just for today.

It's for the coming years of your life.

**What to do today**

- Move multiple times throughout the day

- Don't seek intensity
- Seek frequency
- Integrate movement

**What to avoid today**

- ❌ Thinking only exercise "counts"
- ❌ Sitting all day
- ❌ Forcing yourself into routines you hate
- ❌ Seeing movement as punishment

**Well-integrated movement adds up without draining you.**

**What to focus on**

- Naturalness
- Flow
- Frictionless consistency

Today, your body begins to feel active by nature—
not by obligation.

**Before closing the day**

**Burn this in:**

- An active body sustains itself
- Daily movement is accumulated health
- Living actively is the simplest way to take care of yourself

**Tomorrow, we'll enter a crucial point:**
**real self-control—**
**when you no longer depend on constant monitoring.**

# 29

# DAY 26 – REAL SELF-CONTROL

When you no longer force yourself... you simply choose better

For years, self-control was presented as a constant battle.

Resisting. Enduring. Saying no.

Fighting yourself over and over again.

That approach is exhausting.

And what exhausts you eventually gets abandoned.

This chapter exists to teach you something very different:

Real self-control is not force.

It is clarity.

When there is clarity, choosing well becomes natural.

Today's goal

- Redefine the concept of self-control
- Eliminate constant monitoring
- Consolidate automatic, conscious decisions

**Today, we don't train resistance.**

**Today, we consolidate inner mastery.**

**1️⃣ False self-control (and why it always fails)**

**False self-control looks like this:**

- rigid prohibitions
- constant mental struggle
- fear of "losing control"
- emotional exhaustion

**This type of control depends on mental energy.**

**And mental energy runs out.**

**When it runs out, excess appears.**

**2️⃣ Real self-control is born from coherence**

**True self-control doesn't shout.**

**It doesn't tighten.**

**It doesn't threaten.**

**It works because:**

- you eat well most of the time
- you move regularly
- you sleep better
- you reduce stress

**When the body is regulated, the mind doesn't panic.**

**And when there is no panic, there is control.**

**3️⃣ Choosing well without overthinking**

**Notice something important:**

**When you're aligned:**

- you don't need to negotiate as much
- you don't need to justify yourself
- you don't need "willpower"

**You simply choose.**

**Not because you force yourself—**

**but because you no longer want to sabotage yourself.**

**That's the moment when self-control becomes quiet.**

**4 The mistake of monitoring yourself when it's no longer necessary**

**Many people keep monitoring themselves out of fear.**

They think:

*"If I stop controlling myself, everything will fall apart."*

**That belief creates unnecessary tension.**

**Excessive monitoring breaks trust.**

**And without trust, the system weakens.**

**Today, we begin to release that monitoring—**
**without losing structure.**

**5 Self-control is not denying yourself pleasure**

**Denying pleasure creates rebound.**

**Real self-control looks like this:**

- you choose when
- you choose how much
- you choose why

**You don't eat on impulse.**

**You eat by decision.**

**That changes everything.**

**6 When self-control becomes identity**

**There comes a point where you no longer say:**

*"I have to control myself."*

**You begin to live as:**

*"This is who I am now."*

**And when behavior integrates into identity,**
**it no longer requires effort.**

**That's the level you're reaching.**

**What to do today**

- Trust your decisions
- Maintain core habits
- Reduce unnecessary monitoring
- Choose calmly

**What to avoid today**

- ❌ Controlling yourself out of fear
- ❌ Prohibiting yourself out of anxiety
- ❌ Thinking control means rigidity
- ❌ Constantly doubting yourself

**Real self-control doesn't feel tense.**

**What to focus on**

- Clarity
- Trust
- Inner mastery

**Today, you're no longer fighting yourself.**

**You're aligned.**

**Before closing the day**

**Burn this in deeply:**

- Self-control is not imposed
- It is built
- And when it's built, it liberates

**Tomorrow, we enter the final stretch:**

**preparing for the future—**

**where the process no longer has an end date.**

# 30

# DAY 27 – PREPARING FOR THE FUTURE

When the process no longer has an expiration date

If you've made it this far, one thing is undeniable:

This stopped being a challenge.

It became a way of living.

And precisely because of that, this chapter is crucial.

Many people achieve temporary changes...

but fail when the process "ends."

This book was not designed to end.

It was designed to continue with you.

Today's goal

- Stop thinking in terms of "after the plan"
- Build a long-term vision
- Mentally prepare yourself to maintain results without fear

Today, we don't close anything.

Today, we open the future.

1️⃣ The mistake of thinking the process ends

**One of the most common thoughts is this:**

*"What do I do once this is over?"*

**That question already contains the problem.**

**Because it assumes:**

- change is temporary
- the system shuts down
- "normal life" returns

**Here, we establish a different truth:**

**You don't go back to your old life.**

**You evolve into a new normal.**

**2️⃣ The future isn't improvised—it's designed**

**The body doesn't maintain itself by accident.**

**It maintains itself through repeated decisions over time.**

**You don't need a rigid plan forever.**

**You need clear principles.**

**Principles such as:**

- eating with awareness
- moving regularly
- resting better
- adjusting when necessary

**These principles don't expire.**

**3️⃣ Thinking in stages, not endings**

**Life moves in stages:**

- more structured weeks
- more flexible weeks
- periods of higher demand
- periods of recovery

**Thinking in stages allows you to:**

- adapt without guilt
- adjust without quitting
- continue without drama

**The mistake is thinking in black and white.**

**4 The mindset of conscious maintenance**

**Maintaining is not resisting.**

**Maintaining is living aligned.**

**When you see maintenance as heavy, you avoid it.**

**When you understand it as basic coherence, it becomes natural.**

**Today, we install this idea:**

**Maintaining is easier than starting over.**

**And you already know that.**

**5 Preparing for difficult moments**

**There will be weeks:**

- with more stress
- with less time
- with more pressure

**That doesn't break the process.**

**What breaks it is not anticipating it.**

**Prepare yourself with this mindset:**

- in hard weeks, lower expectations
- maintain minimum habits
- don't quit
- return fully when you can

**That way of thinking makes you resilient.**

**6 The future belongs to those who don't quit**

**Here is the final truth of this chapter:**

**You don't win by doing it perfectly.**

**You win by continuing.**

**And you've already learned how to continue.**

**What to do today**

- Visualize your life with this system fully integrated
- Think in principles, not rules
- Reinforce core habits
- Maintain perspective

**What to avoid today**

- ❌ Thinking in terms of "ending"
- ❌ Fearing the future
- ❌ Believing you'll need to start over
- ❌ Underestimating what you've built

**The future doesn't intimidate you.**

**It belongs to you.**

**What to focus on**

- Continuity
- Vision
- Long-term stability

**Today, you're not closing a plan.**

**You're securing a way of living.**

**Before closing the day**

**Burn this in deeply:**

- The process doesn't end
- It evolves with you
- And you already know how to adapt

**Tomorrow, we enter the emotional final stretch:**

**Day 28 – Closing the Process,**

where everything you've built gets sealed.

# 31

# DAY 28 – CLOSING THE PROCESS

**You didn't finish a plan. You became someone new.**

If you made it this far, there's something no one can take from you:

**Proof that you can sustain yourself.**

Not because you were perfect—

but because you didn't quit.

This chapter doesn't exist to say goodbye to the process.

It exists so you understand what just happened inside you.

Because what changed wasn't only your body.

It was the way you decide.

The way you continue.

The way you see yourself.

**Today's goal**

- Recognize the full transformation
- Close the process without letting go of what you built
- Integrate what you've learned as a permanent identity

Today, we don't celebrate through excess.

Today, we recognize with clarity.

1️⃣ **It wasn't the weight. It was coherence.**

If you lost weight, excellent.

If you lost less than you expected, that's fine too.

Because the most important thing was never the number.

It was that you:

- learned not to quit
- stopped punishing yourself
- understood your body
- built real habits

That matters more than any figure.

The body always catches up to an aligned mind.

2️⃣ **The real win: you no longer depend on "starting over"**

Before, you needed:

- Monday
- a new month
- motivation
- "this time for real"

Not anymore.

Now you know:

**you don't need to start over—you just need to continue.**

That truth frees you from endless cycles.

3️⃣ **Who you were vs. who you are now**

No drama. No exaggeration. Just truth.

**Before:**

- you doubted
- you demanded too much of yourself
- you gave up easily
- you lived in extremes

**Now:**

- you adjust
- you continue
- you trust
- you sustain

That change is irreversible.

### 4 The mistake you must NOT make now

Here is the final warning:

❌ Don't think this was just "a challenge you completed."

❌ Don't walk away from what works.

❌ Don't test yourself by returning to chaos.

Not because you're weak—

but because you no longer need it.

The system already lives inside you.

### 5 The process is internal now

From this point forward:

- you don't depend on the book
- you don't depend on the calendar
- you don't depend on daily structure

You depend on principles.

And principles don't expire.

You already know:

- how to adjust
- how to continue
- how to return
- how to take care of yourself

That is mastery.

### 6 A closing that doesn't feel like an ending

This process doesn't end with the word "finish."

It ends with something far more powerful:

**A new normal.**

Eating better no longer feels like effort.

Moving no longer feels like punishment.

Taking care of yourself no longer feels like a fight.

It's who you are.

**What to do today**

- Acknowledge your full process
- Appreciate your consistency
- Maintain the core habits
- Continue—without drama

**What to avoid today**

- ❌ Seeking external validation
- ❌ Comparing yourself
- ❌ Thinking you need something more
- ❌ Underestimating what you achieved

What you built is already enough.

**What to focus on**

- Identity
- Continuity
- Real life

Today, you're not closing a book.

You're closing a chapter of struggle.

**Before you close this chapter (and this cycle)**

Burn this in, because it's the final truth:

- It wasn't luck
- It wasn't motivation
- It was sustained coherence

And that... no one can ever take from you.

PART III

# MAINTENANCE & LIFESTYLE INTEGRATION

## Where the Result Becomes Permanent

If you've made it this far, you've already accomplished what most people never do:

you didn't quit.

But now comes something even more important.

Losing weight is not the real challenge.

The real challenge is not going back.

And that is not achieved through more willpower,

more rules,

or living in fear.

It's achieved through identity, judgment, and lifestyle.

This section of the book exists to answer the questions most people never learn how to answer:

- How do I maintain my results without living on a diet?
- What do I do when there is no longer a daily plan?

• How do I avoid rebound without rigidity or anxiety?

• Who do I need to become so I don't lose what I've gained?

Here, we leave behind the concept of a "30-day plan" and step into a way of living.

**This Part Doesn't Ask You to Do More**

**It Asks You to Understand Better**

Up to this point, you followed a clear structure.

That was necessary.

But real life doesn't work in numbered days.

It works through repeated decisions,

through judgment,

through identity.

In this section, you'll learn how to:

- Maintain results without fear
- Adjust without sabotaging yourself
- Live with intelligent flexibility
- Consolidate an identity that does not rebound

There are no extremes here.

No punishment.

No backtracking.

There is physical and mental maturity.

**The Mistake This Section Prevents**

Many people lose weight...

and then gain it all back because they:

- Stop paying attention
- Return to old patterns
- Believe "it's over"
- Disconnect from what they learned

This section exists so that doesn't happen to you.

Not because you're weak.

But because maintenance requires awareness, not effort.

**What You'll Find in the Next Chapters**

In the chapters ahead, you'll learn:

- How to keep the weight off, even during difficult phases
- What to do after the 30 days, without losing direction
- The identity of someone who stays in shape, so results feel natural—not forced

These chapters won't give you new rules.

They'll give you judgment.

And when you have judgment,

you don't need anyone watching over you.

**Before You Continue**

Understand this with absolute clarity:

You are not defending a result.

You are consolidating a version of yourself.

And when the version changes,

the result maintains itself.

Take a breath.

Turn the page.

This is where the change becomes permanent.

32

# HOW NOT TO REGAIN THE WEIGHT

## The real reason most people go back... and how to prevent it forever

Regaining the weight isn't a personal failure.

It's a failure of approach.

Most people believe they regain weight because they "relaxed,"

because they "let themselves go,"

or because they "lost discipline."

The truth is simpler... and more uncomfortable:

They regain the weight because they never changed the way they live.

This chapter exists to make sure that never happens to you.

### The goal of this chapter

- Understand why rebound happens long term

- Eliminate the invisible mistakes that cause it
- Build a structure that maintains itself without effort

We're not adding new rules here.

We're fixing the foundation.

### 1 Rebound doesn't start with food

Rebound almost never starts with what you eat.

It starts with what you stop doing.

It shows up like this:

- less daily movement
- less rest
- more stress
- less awareness

Food is only the final reflection.

When the foundation weakens, the body goes back into protection mode.

### 2 The fatal mistake: going back to "normal life"

After a successful process, many people think:

"Now I can go back to my normal life."

But that "normal life" is what created the original problem.

Here we establish a clear truth:

You don't go back to your old life.

You evolve into a new normal.

That doesn't mean living restricted.

It means living more consciously.

### 3 Emotional rebound (the one no one sees coming)

Before the weight returns, what often shows up first is:

- mental neglect
- "I'll get back to it later"
- improvising
- losing presence

The body follows the mind.
When the mind disconnects, the body follows.

**4 THE RULE that protects everything**

Store this as a personal law:
Never break all your habits at the same time.
If one day you eat worse:

- move
- sleep
- hydrate

If one week is chaotic:

- keep the minimum
- don't quit

Rebound happens when everything breaks.

**5 WEIGHT ISN'T MAINTAINED through constant monitoring—it's maintained through identity**

Monitoring yourself forever isn't realistic.
The right question isn't:
"How do I control myself?"
It's:
"Who am I now?"
When your identity changes:

- your decisions change
- your habits align
- your weight stabilizes

This book helped you change your identity.

This chapter teaches you how to protect it.

### 6 What to do when **life gets complicated**

There will be phases:

- with more stress
- with less time
- with less energy

That doesn't break the process.

The right strategy is:

- lower expectations
- maintain the core habits
- return fully when you can

Flexible consistency beats rigid perfection.

### 7 The mindset **that prevents rebound forever**

The right mindset is this:

- not "I failed"
- not "I fell off"
- not "I'll start over"

The right phrase is:

"I adjust and I continue."

And you continue.

That's it.

### What to do **from now on**

- Protect your core habits
- Adjust without quitting
- Stay present
- Live from your new normal

. . .

**What to avoid at all costs**

- ✖ Going back to autopilot
- ✖ Thinking "it's over"
- ✖ Breaking everything because of one mistake
- ✖ Living in fear of rebound

Fear creates tension.

Tension creates rebound.

**What to focus on**

- Awareness
- Stability
- Identity

Today you're not protecting a result.

You're protecting who you are now.

**Chapter closing**

Burn this in deeply:

Weight isn't maintained through sacrifice.

It's maintained through coherence.

And coherence... already lives in you.

# 33

# WHAT TO DO AFTER THE 30 DAYS

## When There's No Daily Plan — And That's Exactly the Point

Reaching the end of a plan often creates a quiet, dangerous question:

**"So... what do I do now?"**

That single question has sabotaged more results than any meal, any mistake, or any difficult week ever could.

Because when someone believes the plan is over,

the body and the mind start waiting to go back.

This chapter exists to make one thing absolutely clear:

**There is no "after" the process.**

**There is only a freer, more conscious, more mature continuation.**

### The Purpose of This Chapter

- To remove dependence on a daily plan

- To teach you how to live without rigid instructions
- To turn what you've learned into permanent judgment

This chapter does not tell you what to do every day.

**It teaches you how to decide.**

### 1 The Mistake of Immediately Looking for Another Plan

When people finish a process, many immediately look for:

- another challenge
- another diet
- another program
- another rigid structure

Not because they need it.

**Because they don't trust themselves yet.**

Searching for another plan too quickly is often a way to avoid responsibility.

Today, we do the opposite.

**We trust what you've already built.**

### 2 Real Change Doesn't Require Constant Instructions

If over these 30 days you learned how to:

- eat with awareness
- move consistently
- rest better
- adjust without quitting

Then you no longer need someone telling you exactly what to do.

What you need now is **judgment**.

And judgment looks like this:

- you make better choices most of the time

• you adjust when things drift
• you continue without drama

That is physical and mental maturity.

### 3 How to Structure Life Without a "Day 1"

Life does not work in perfect cycles.
It works in real weeks.
A simple and powerful structure is this:

• **Daily base habits**
(mindful eating, movement, hydration, rest)
• **Weekly flexibility**
(events, changes, imperfect days)
• **Periodic review**
(not daily, not obsessive)

You don't need more than that.

### 4 What to Do When You Feel Like You're "Slipping"

This is a critical skill.
When you notice that:

• you're eating worse
• you're moving less
• things feel slightly off

Don't panic.
Don't dramatize.
Do this:

1 Acknowledge it
2 Adjust one thing
3 Continue

**Never restart from zero.**
That belongs to the old mindset.

. . .

### 5 Weight Is No Longer the Center of the Process

After the 30 days, weight stops being the main character.

What matters more now is:

- how you feel
- how you decide
- how you sustain yourself
- how you adapt

Weight becomes a secondary outcome, not an obsession.

And that is freedom.

### 6 When to Repeat a Structured Phase

There will be moments when you want to:

- refocus
- reorganize habits
- raise your level of discipline

It's perfectly fine to return to more structured phases — **with awareness, not desperation.**

The difference is this:

You're no longer doing it because you're lost.

You're doing it because you know exactly where you're going.

### 7 The Final Sign That the Process Worked

The real sign isn't your body.

It's this internal sentence:

**"I know what to do when things get off track."**

When you have that,

you no longer depend on books, plans, or challenges.

You depend on yourself.

. . .

### What to Do From Now On

- Live from your base habits
- Adjust without fear
- Continue without drama
- Trust your judgment

### What to Avoid

- ❌ Unnecessary rigidity
- ❌ Thinking you need to "start over"
- ❌ Waiting for the "perfect plan"
- ❌ Returning to unconscious autopilot

Your autopilot now works in your favor.

### What to Focus On

- Coherence
- Judgment
- Conscious continuity

You're not finishing a process.

**You're starting to live from what you've learned.**

### Chapter Close

Etch this deeply into your mind:

**You don't need another plan.**

**You need to trust the person you've become.**

And that person...

**already knows how to maintain results.**

# 34

# THE IDENTITY OF A PERSON WHO STAYS IN SHAPE

## The Identity of a Person Who Stays in Shape

**It's Not What You Do. It's Who You Are.**

Most people believe that staying in shape requires constant effort.

Endless vigilance.

Permanent sacrifice.

That's why they live tired.

That's why they live in fear.

And that's why, sooner or later, they return to where they started.

The truth is different:

**People who stay in shape don't rely on willpower.**

**They live from a different identity.**

This chapter exists so that identity becomes yours.

### The Real Change Was Never Physical

If you only change your body, the change is fragile.

If you change your identity, the body follows naturally.

People who stay in shape:

- don't "fight" food
- don't "force themselves" to move
- don't live in punishment mode

They simply don't live the way they used to.

And that changes everything.

### Who Is a Person Who Truly Stays in Shape?

Not someone perfect.

Not someone rigid.

Not someone obsessive.

It's someone who:

- takes care of themselves without drama
- adjusts without guilt
- continues without excuses
- respects themselves without punishment

Physical shape is a consequence.

Not a daily battle.

### Identity Is Revealed in Small Decisions

Identity is not proven on perfect days.

It's revealed on ordinary ones.

In decisions like:

- eating with awareness even when no one is watching
- moving even when motivation is low
- resting without guilt
- adjusting without quitting

That's where real identity lives.

. . .

### The Difference Between "Defending" and "Maintaining"

Defending a body is exhausting.

Maintaining it is natural.

When you feel like you have to "defend yourself" from food,

from social events,

from life itself...

the identity is not solid yet.

But when you choose well without fighting,

when you adjust without fear,

when you enjoy without losing yourself...

you're no longer defending anything.

You're living from who you are.

### A Person Who Stays in Shape Thinks Differently

They don't think:

- "I broke the diet"
- "I failed"
- "I'll start on Monday"

They think:

- "I adjust today"
- "I continue tomorrow"
- "This is part of my life"

That internal dialogue is what sustains the result.

### Identity Doesn't Disappear During Difficult Times

There will be stages:

- with stress
- with fatigue
- with limited time

The old version quit.
The new version adjusts.
No drama.
No punishment.
No going backward.
They understand that coherence isn't measured in days
—
it's measured in trajectories.

## The Body Responds to the Dominant Identity

The body doesn't respond to promises.
It responds to patterns.
When your identity is:
**"I'm someone who takes care of myself,"**
the body:

- regulates appetite
- cooperates with movement
- adapts to its environment

Not because you force it.
Because you support it with consistency.

## The Final Identity (Read This Slowly)

A person who stays in shape:

- doesn't chase shortcuts
- doesn't live in extremes
- doesn't need constant monitoring
- doesn't depend on motivation

They live with awareness.
They adjust when necessary.
They continue without drama.
And that...

**changes everything.**

### The True Closing of This Book

This book was not written so you would follow it forever.

It was written so you would no longer need it.

Because now you know:

- how to take care of yourself
- how to adjust
- how to maintain
- how to continue

And when you know who you are,
you no longer need constant instructions.

### Final Words (The Most Important Ones)

Etch this deeply into your mind, because it is the final truth:

**You are not in shape because you follow a plan.**

**You stay in shape because this is who you are now.**

And a well-built identity
**is never lost.**

## THIS WASN'T A BOOK. IT WAS A DECISION.

You can no longer say you don't know.

You can no longer say "this isn't for me."

You can no longer say "it's always the same."

Because now you have evidence.

Not promises.

Not theory.

**Lived evidence.**

This book didn't change you.

It showed you what you're capable of when you stop quitting.

**It Wasn't Force. It Was Coherence.**

You didn't lose weight because you suffered.

You didn't change because you punished yourself.

You didn't maintain results because you monitored yourself endlessly.

You changed because:

- you observed yourself
- you adjusted

- you continued
- you trusted

That is maturity.
That is power.

### The Real Achievement Isn't Visible in the Mirror

The mirror shows a reflection.
But the real change lives somewhere else.
It lives in:

- how you think when things fall out of order
- how you decide when no one is watching
- how you continue when motivation is gone
- how you respect yourself without punishment

That is what sustains you.

### From Today On, You're No Longer "Trying"

From today on:

- you're not starting
- you're not experimenting
- you're not waiting

You are living from a different identity.
And identity is not negotiated on difficult days.
It is adjusted.
It is protected.
It is honored.

### This Book Doesn't End Here

This book ends when you no longer need it.
When decisions come naturally.
When the body cooperates.

When chaos no longer drags you back.
And if one day you doubt,
if one day you stumble,
if one day life tightens its grip...
Don't start over.
**Continue.**
That's all.

### The Final Truth (Read This Twice)

It wasn't luck.

It wasn't genetics.

It wasn't motivation.

It was a repeated decision.

And now you know something very few people ever learn:

**The body changes when identity changes.**
**And the identity you've built...**
**does not disappear.**
**— Edgar Hernández**

# MEET THE AUTHOR: THE FOUNDER OF INSPIRED LEGACY PRESS

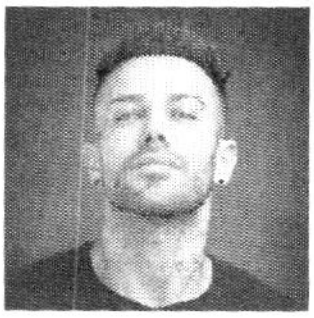

**Edgar Hernández** is an author, speaker, and architect of human transformation. He is the founder of **Inspired Legacy Press**, an independent publishing imprint through which he leads a global movement dedicated to the mastery and evolution of human potential.

His work integrates **philosophy, science, and behavioral psychology** with emotional intelligence, neurobiohacking, performance biology, longevity science, high-level habits, and systematic physical development to cultivate **mental clarity, inner strength, and unbreakable discipline.**

He is the creator of the **Inspired Legacy Framework**, a system of human transformation built upon four dimensions: **identity, body, wealth, and spirit.**

This framework is designed for individuals who choose to forge character, master their vital energy, expand their awareness, and build a life defined by real results rather than temporary motivation.

Through his books and teachings, he maintains a central conviction:

**Those who master their mind, their emotions, and their habits... master their destiny.**

This book forms part of an **Editorial System** conceived for the integral transformation of the individual.

A system built upon principles, structure, and long-term vision, where each work fulfills a precise role within a greater whole: cultivating **mental clarity, self-discipline, inner strength, and a conscious identity** capable of sustaining real results across the four dimensions of human development—**identity, body, wealth, and spirit.**

The purpose of the **Inspired Editorial System** is to refine judgment, elevate thinking, and forge character.

Each book is a pillar.

Each concept is a tool for real life.

This system is intended for those who understand that **personal growth is not a trend, but a deliberate and structured practice**—that freedom is built through knowledge, decision, and coherence—and that every true legacy begins in **the architecture of the mind.**

**This is not self-help.**

**This is human architecture.**

**Master your identity.**

**Strengthen your body.**

**Multiply your wealth.**

**Expand your spirit.**

**Build power.**

**Build freedom.**

**Build legacy.**

**Welcome to the Inspired Universe.**

Printed in Dunstable, United Kingdom

91342778R00100